MRCP PART 1
MCQ PRACTICE EXAMS
Second Edition

D0726675

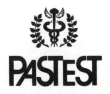

PASTEST

MRCP PART 1
MCQ PRACTICE EXAMS
Second Edition

Compiled and edited by

Malcolm Littley MD MRCP
Consultant Physician,
Burnley Healthcare NHS Trust,
Lancashire.

First edition 1982
Updated 1989
Second edition 1995
Reprinted 1996

ISBN: 0 906896 49 5

A catalogue record for this book is available from the British Library.

Typeset by Editext, Knutsford, Cheshire.
Printed by BPC Wheatons, Exeter.

CONTENTS

PASTEST INTENSIVE COURSES FOR MRCP PART 1

For over 22 years PasTest, the leading independent specialists in postgraduate medical education, have been delivering top quality courses which have helped many thousands of doctors to pass the demanding MRCP Part 1 examination.

PasTest MRCP Part 1 courses are

- ✓ Intensive, practical and exam oriented
- ✓ Designed to strengthen exam technique
- ✓ Interactive and entertaining
- ✓ The key to exam success

Our reputation is built on results. With the official Royal College pass rate at 35%, PasTest delegates consistently achieve a pass rate of well over 60%. This is a competitive edge that you cannot afford to ignore.

Our six-day MRCP Part 1 revision courses run three times each year at a convenient central London venue. Each delegate receives detailed course notes consisting of approximately 250 pages of exam-based MCQs with answers and comprehensive notes, plus many explanatory handouts.

- ✓ Learn from experienced and talented tutors with up-to-date knowledge of the requirements of the exam

- ✓ Teaching sessions focus on "favourite" exam topics and highlight possible areas of difficulty

- ✓ Four full practice exams enable you to constantly monitor your performance as the course progresses

For full details of the range of PasTest books and courses available for MRCP Part 1 candidates, contact PasTest today:

**PasTest, Dept. PEB, Egerton Court, Parkgate Estate,
Knutsford, Cheshire WA16 8DX
Telephone 01565 755226   Fax 01565 650264**

EDITOR'S NOTE

This new edition has been published at a time of great change in medicine and in the Membership examination. The increased emphasis on basic science and the separation of the adult and paediatric examinations has brought about the need for a complete revision of subject material.

Most of the advances in medicine are being made in the area of basic science and are incorporated very rapidly into daily clinical practice. Some parts of this book are unashamedly up to date, particularly in this area. This reflects the need to provide a book which is 'future-proof' for at least a few years!

The answers and explanations in this edition are more comprehensive than in previous editions. It is hoped that this will help candidates to have a broader understanding of the subject area concerned and that the information will help them to pass the exam, as well as guiding them in clinical practice. However, it should be emphasized that reading the recommended texts is an essential part of the learning process.

Finally, I am indebted to the large number of doctors around the country (listed overleaf) who have contributed to this book in their own subject area. Without them, none of this would have been possible. This is testament to the continuing commitment of the medical profession to postgraduate education.

Malcolm Littley MD MRCP
Consultant Physician
Burnley Healthcare NHS Trust

ACKNOWLEDGEMENTS

The Editor wishes to thank the following doctors for their contributions to this book:

Dr Richard Bull, Senior Registrar, Department of Dermatology, The Royal London Hospital.

Dr E. Brian Faragher, Medical Statistician, Department of Medical Statistics, Withington Hospital, Manchester.

Dr Iain Fraser, Research Registrar, Department of Infectious Diseases and Tropical Medicine, North Manchester General Hospital.

Dr Jane Hamilton, Senior Registrar, University Department of Psychiatry, Manchester Royal Infirmary.

Dr Andrew D. Higham, MRC Clinical Training Fellow, Honorary Senior Registrar, Department of Medicine, Section of Gastroenterology, Hope Hospital, Salford.

Dr Simon Jowitt, Senior Registrar in Haematology, North West Regional Rotation.

Dr Phil Kalra, Consultant Nephrologist, Hope Hospital, Salford.

Dr Christopher Marguerie, Consultant Physician, Department of Medicine, Warwick Hospital.

Dr Donal J. O'Donoghue, Consultant Renal Physician, Department of Renal Medicine, Salford Royal Hospitals NHS Trust.

Dr Stephen Owen, Consultant Physician in Respiratory Medicine, Warrington Hospital, Cheshire.

Dr Martin Pattrick, Consultant Physician and Rheumatologist, North Manchester General Hospital.

Dr Nicholas S. Peters, Senior Lecturer and Honorary Consultant, Department of Cardiology, St. Mary's Hospital, London.

Dr Andrew Scott, Senior Lecturer in Geriatric Medicine, Department of Geriatric Medicine, University of Manchester, Hope Hospital.

Dr Paul R. Talbot, Senior Registrar in Department of Neurology, Manchester Royal Infirmary.

Dr Edmund Wilkins, Consultant Physician Infectious Diseases, Monsall Unit, North Manchester General Hospital.

INTRODUCTION

The MRCP Part 1 is a highly competitive examination. There is no fixed pass mark, instead there is a fixed pass *rate* of 35%. This means that 65% of candidates must fail the examination. To pass the exam you must outshine your colleagues. PasTest revision books and courses are designed to give ambitious candidates a competitive edge.

Multiple choice questions are the most reliable and consistent method we have of testing re-call of factual knowledge. A well designed MCQ paper can assess candidates' understanding of basic facts, principles, concepts and reasoning ability. The most important function of an MCQ paper of the type used in the MRCP Part 1 examination is to rank candidates accurately and fairly according to their performance.

How to use this book

Before you take one of the Practice Exams in this book, read the revision checklists at the beginning of the book and make sure that you feel confident that you have covered these important topics. PasTest publish a number of books which contain MCQs suitable for MRCP Part 1 arranged by subject, and these can help you to identify and iron out any particular weaknesses. If you need to read up on any subject, check the reading list at the back of this book for advice. With time at a premium, it is best to concentrate on the most important subjects covered in the exam. It is unlikely that there will be more than one question covering statistics, genetics or ophthalmology in each exam paper, so plan your revision accordingly.

To make the best use of these Practice Exams you should take them under strict timed conditions, allowing 2½ hours for each paper. Correct your answers carefully and read the explanations to the answers. These notes are a reminder of the most important points on each topic and provide guidance on areas which candidates are most likely to find difficult.

Reasons for getting an answer wrong include poor knowledge, memory at fault, misunderstood the question, hasty/wild guess. It is important for you to understand why you got a question wrong so that you can learn from your mistakes.

Exam technique

There are two common mistakes which cause good candidates to fail the MRCP Part 1. These are failing to read the directions and questions carefully enough, and failing to fill in the computer answer card properly.

Introduction

You must read the question (both stem and items) carefully. Regard each item as being independent of every other item, each refers to a specific quantum of knowledge. The item (or the stem and the item taken together) make up a statement. You are required to indicate whether you regard this statement as "True" or "False", and you are also able to indicate that you "Don't Know". A system of negative marking is used. For every correct answer you gain a mark (+1) and for every incorrect answer you lose a mark (−1). No marks are awarded for indicating "Don't Know".

Look only at each single statement when answering, and disregard all the other parts of the question. They have nothing to do with the item you are concentrating on.

The answer sheet is read by an automatic document reader, which transfers the information it reads to a computer. It is critical that the answer sheet is filled in clearly and accurately using the pencils provided. Failure to fill in your name and your examination correctly could result in rejection of your paper.

You need to decide on your own personal strategy for approaching the paper. Some candidates mark their answers on the computer sheet as they go through the questions, others prefer to make a note of their answers on the question paper, and then reserve time at the end to transfer their answers to the computer sheet. If you choose the first method, there is a chance that you may decide to change your answer after a second reading. If you do change an answer, be sure that your original mark is thoroughly erased. If you choose the second method, make sure that you do allow enough time to transfer your answers methodically onto the computer sheet as rushing at this stage could introduce some costly mistakes.

Some candidates try to calculate their scores as they work through the paper; their theory is that if they reach a certain score they should then be safe in indicating "Don't Know" for any items they have left blank without needing to take the trouble to think out the answers. This is a dangerous game to play, as you cannot be sure of your score. Furthermore, since the exam is based on a pass *rate* rather than a pass *mark*, you cannot be sure of the mark you will need to achieve in order to be included in the top 35% of candidates. A safer rule of thumb is that you will probably need to answer between 230–250 items to gain enough marks to pass.

There are 60 questions to complete in 2½ hours. This works out at 25 minutes for 10 questions. Most candidates find that they have more than enough time and there can be a temptation to re-read your answers time and time again until even those that seemed straightforward start to look less convincing. In this situation, first thoughts are usually best. Don't be afraid to leave the examination room once you are satisfied with your answers.

To guess or not to guess

Tests carried out at PasTest's MRCP Part 1 intensive revision courses have proved that by far the majority of candidates can improve their marks by making sensible educated guesses. Most candidates fail the exam by a very few marks and becoming a good guesser can give you the extra boost that you need to rise above the average.

Where there is any chance that you can reach the answer by drawing on first principles and your reasoning power, then it is worth making an educated guess.

If you feel that you need to spend more time puzzling over a question, leave it and, if you have time, return to it. Make sure you have collected all the marks you can before you come back to any difficult questions.

If you really have no idea about the answer, then a lucky guess might gain you a mark, but there is an equal chance that you will lose a mark. In this case, do not guess. Use the "Don't Know" option.

Final advice

Multiple choice questions are not designed to trick you or confuse you, they are designed to test your knowledge of medicine. Accept each question at its face value, do not look for hidden meanings or catches.

The aim of this book is to enable you to evaluate your level of knowledge by working through five mock Membership examination papers. By marking clearly all the questions that you got wrong or declined to answer you can then refresh your memory with the explanations given here or read up on the specific topic in depth using a textbook.

Working through these exams will help you to identify your weak subject areas. You must work out your own personal profile of strengths and weaknesses and plan your revision accordingly. In the last few weeks before the exam it will be important for you to concentrate on the most important subject areas covered in the exam.

A breakdown of the relative distribution of topics in the exam is given below. Variations may occur from exam to exam.

Subject area	Number of MCQs
Neurology	5/6
Clinical Pharmacology/Toxicology	5/6
Basic Sciences	5/6
Cardiology	4/5
Gastroenterology	4/5
Respiratory Medicine	4/5
Infectious disease/AIDS/Tropical Med	4
Endocrinology	4
Rheumatology/Immunology	4
Nephrology	4
Psychiatry	3
Haematology	3
Metabolism	2/3
Dermatology	1
Statistics	1
Genetics	1
Geriatrics	1
Ophthalmology	1
Total number of MCQs	60

For last minute revision the MCQs in this book have been categorised under subjects on page 141. Thus, a quick review of cardiology or neurology is possible by running through all the MCQs in this book that fall under this heading.

Finally, the best approach to the exam is to ensure that your knowledge of medicine and its specialties is sound, to answer each exam question to the best of your ability, and to make every possible effort to work out the answers to the more difficult questions.

Good luck on the day.

REVISION CHECKLISTS

This list is not intended to be exhaustive and should not be regarded as a syllabus for the examination. However, it represents the subject areas covered in recent examinations and a selection of topics identified by our course lecturers as being essential background knowledge. These subjects are therefore likely to be encountered in the exam and your revision should cover most if not all of these subjects. Some subjects require more detailed knowledge than others, but practice questions should help you to find the correct level. Tick off the box against each topic as you cover it in your revision sessions and it will help you to target the most important areas as your exam draws nearer.

CARDIOLOGY

Basic science/physiology/anatomy
☐ JVP waveform
☐ Embryology of heart and great vessels
☐ Action potential
☐ ECG physiology
☐ Anterior mediastinal contents

Clinical disorders/pathophysiology/complications
☐ Pericarditis
☐ Cardiomyopathy
☐ Congenital heart disease
☐ Congenital cause of arrhythmia
☐ Ischaemic heart disease
☐ Myocardial infarction
☐ Valvular heart disease
☐ Infective endocarditis
☐ Supraventricular tachycardia
☐ Ventricular tachycardia
☐ Bradyarrhythmias
☐ Hypertension

Investigation
☐ Electrolyte disorders and the ECG
☐ Echocardiography

Therapy
☐ Thrombolysis
☐ Anti-arrhythmic agents
☐ Anti-hypertensive agents
☐ Anti-anginal agents

DIABETES AND METABOLISM

Basic science/physiology/anatomy
- [ ] Acid base balance, anion gap ✔
- [ ] Oxygen dissociation curve ✔
- [ ] Lipoprotein metabolism
- [ ] Plasma proteins, enzymes

Clinical disorders/pathophysiology/complications
- [ ] IDDM vs NIDDM clinical features ✔
- [ ] Acute complications (e.g. DKA, hypoglycaemia) ✔
- [ ] Microvascular complications ✔
- [ ] Spontaneous hypoglycaemia ✔
- [ ] Electrolyte disorders (high or low, Na, K, Ca, etc) ✔
- [ ] Vitamin deficiency/excess ✔
- [ ] Rare disorders (e.g. Wilson's, haemochromatosis) ✔
- [ ] Porphyria (especially AIP and PCT) ✔
- [ ] Metabolic response to trauma ✔
- [ ] Hypothermia ✔
- [ ] Ethanol excess ✔
- [ ] Environmental and drug poisoning ✔
- [ ] Parathyroid, vitamin D, calcium regulation ✔
- [ ] Bone disease (e.g. Paget's, osteoporosis) ✔
- [ ] Rhabdomyolysis ✔

Investigation
- [ ] Lipoprotein profiles, categorization
- [ ] Haemoglobin A1c ✔
- [ ] Microalbuminuria ✔
- [ ] Parathyroid and PTH-rP ✔
- [ ] Electrolyte/acid-base features (of e.g. ureterosigmoidostomy) ✔

Therapy
- [ ] Oral hypoglycaemic action ✔
- [ ] Lipid lowering agents ✔
- [ ] Specific poisoning antidotes ✔

DERMATOLOGY

Basic science/physiology/anatomy
- [ ] Structure of skin
- [ ] Cell types

Clinical disorders/pathophysiology/complications
- ☐ Specific dermatoses (psoriasis, eczema, etc)
- ☐ Skin malignancy
- ☐ Manifestations of systemic disease
- ☐ Drug eruptions
- ☐ Associations of internal malignancy
- ☐ Genetic conditions predisposing to malignancy
- ☐ Inflammatory bowel disease
- ☐ Diabetes mellitus
- ☐ HIV infection
- ☐ Causes of pruritus
- ☐ Blistering conditions
- ☐ Depigmentation/pigmentation

Investigation
- ☐ Immunochemistry

Therapy
- ☐ Antifungals
- ☐ Topical steroids
- ☐ Psoriasis (calcipotriol, PUVA, retinoids)
- ☐ Acne (retinoids, antibiotics)
- ☐ Parasiticides

ENDOCRINOLOGY

Basic science/physiology/anatomy
- ☐ Pituitary anatomy
- ☐ Hormone action
- ☐ Receptors
- ☐ Protein binding
- ☐ Pulsatility/biorhythms
- ☐ New endocrine/autocrine/paracrine factors (e.g. endothelin)

Clinical disorders/pathophysiology/complications
- ☐ Pituitary hypersecretion
- ☐ Hypopituitarism (anterior and posterior)
- ☐ Thyroid nodule and carcinomas
- ☐ Hypo/hyperthyroidism
- ☐ Parathyroid disease
- ☐ Atrial natriuretic factor
- ☐ Hypoadrenalism

- ☐ Conn's and Cushing's
- ☐ 21 hydroxylase deficiency
- ☐ Multiple endocrine neoplasia
- ☐ Syndromes of end-organ resistance
- ☐ Hypogonadism
- ☐ Gynaecomastia
- ☐ Hirsutism
- ☐ Carcinoid syndrome

Investigation
- ☐ Laboratory measurement
- ☐ Suppression tests (suspected hyperfunction)
- ☐ Stimulation tests (suspected hypofunction)

Therapy
- ☐ Acromegaly
- ☐ Prolactinoma
- ☐ Cushing's syndrome
- ☐ Thyrotoxicosis

GASTROENTEROLOGY

Basic science/physiology/anatomy
- ☐ Physiology of stomach, intestine, liver, pancreas
- ☐ Autonomic nerves
- ☐ *Helicobacter pylori*

Clinical disorders/pathophysiology/complications
- ☐ Achalasia
- ☐ Barrett's oesophagus
- ☐ Peptic ulceration
- ☐ Gastric carcinoma
- ☐ Pancreatitis
- ☐ Chronic liver disease/hepatitis
- ☐ Granulomatous liver disease
- ☐ Ascites
- ☐ Encephalopathy
- ☐ Steatorrhoea/malabsorption
- ☐ Gluten sensitive enteropathy
- ☐ Inflammatory bowel disease
- ☐ Colonic polyps/carcinoma
- ☐ Inherited bowel disease

- [ ] Bacterial overgrowth
- [ ] Pseudomembranous colitis
- [ ] AIDS and GI tract
- [ ] Drug induced liver disease

Investigation
- [ ] Schilling test
- [ ] Features of pancreatitis
- [ ] Immunology and haematology in coeliac disease

Therapy
- [ ] Parenteral nutrition
- [ ] *Helicobacter* eradication
- [ ] Steroids in IBD
- [ ] Oesophageal varices (NB octreotide)
- [ ] Drug metabolism and liver
- [ ] Paracetamol poisoning

GENETICS

- [ ] Autosomal dominant list
- [ ] Autosomal recessive list
- [ ] Sex-linked list
- [ ] Chromosomal disorders
- [ ] Pre-natal diagnosis
- [ ] Genetic anticipation
- [ ] Maternal effect
- [ ] Genetic linkage
- [ ] HLA antigens (chromosome 6)

HAEMATOLOGY

Basic science/physiology/anatomy
- [ ] Iron metabolism
- [ ] Clotting factors

Clinical disorders/pathophysiology/complications
- [ ] Haematinic deficiency
- [ ] Causes of macrocytosis
- [ ] Haemolytic anaemia (causes)
- [ ] Haemoglobinopathy
- [ ] Leucoerythroblastic anaemia

- [ ] Leukaemias
- [ ] Lymphomas
- [ ] Myeloma
- [ ] Polycythaemia
- [ ] Anticoagulation/thrombophilia
- [ ] Lupus anticoagulant
- [ ] Common bleeding disorders
- [ ] Aplastic anaemia
- [ ] Paroxysmal nocturnal haemoglobinuria
- [ ] Transfusion associated viral infection

Investigation
- [ ] Blood film
- [ ] Causes of eosinophilia, monocytosis etc
- [ ] Coagulation factors, clotting times
- [ ] Coomb's test

Therapy
- [ ] Leukaemia
- [ ] Growth factors (erythropoeitin, GCSF, etc)

IMMUNOLOGY

Basic science/physiology/anatomy
- [ ] Hypersensitivity reactions (I-IV)
- [ ] Complement system
- [ ] Synthesis of immunoglobulins
- [ ] Prostaglandins
- [ ] Arachidonic acid

Clinical disorders/pathophysiology/complications
- [ ] Immunodeficiency syndromes
- [ ] Hereditary angioedema
- [ ] Amyloidosis

Investigation
- [ ] Autoantibodies
- [ ] Antinuclear antibodies

Therapy
- [ ] Hereditary angioedema
- [ ] Immunoglobulin deficiency

INFECTIOUS DISEASES

Basic science/physiology/anatomy
- ☐ Epidemiology
- ☐ Types of bacteria
- ☐ Types of virus (incl DNA vs RNA)
- ☐ Insect vectors

Clinical disorders/pathophysiology/complications

Virus
- ☐ Infectious mononucleosis
- ☐ Hepatitis A, B, C, D
- ☐ Herpes (encephalitis)
- ☐ CMV
- ☐ Rabies
- ☐ Viral haemorrhagic fevers

Bacteria
- ☐ Syphilis
- ☐ *Neisseria* sp (NB meningococcus)
- ☐ Pertussis
- ☐ *Helicobacter*
- ☐ *Clostridium difficile*

Protozoa
- ☐ *Toxoplasma*
- ☐ *Plasmodium* (malaria)

Amoebae
- ☐ *Legionella*
- ☐ *Chlamydia*
- ☐ Rickettsial disease

Clinical problems
- ☐ Splenectomised patient
- ☐ Congenital infection
- ☐ Toxic shock syndrome
- ☐ Tropical disease
- ☐ HIV seroconversion
- ☐ HIV typical clinical infections
- ☐ HIV and tumours

Investigation
- [ ] CSF findings
- [ ] CD4 count
- [ ] PUO

Therapy
- [ ] Vaccination
- [ ] Antibiotic spectrum
- [ ] Treatment of pneumonia

NEPHROLOGY

Basic science/physiology/anatomy
- [ ] Renal physiology
- [ ] Anatomy of nephron and vasculature
- [ ] Hormone action in kidney

Clinical disorders/pathophysiology/complications
- [ ] Glomerulonephritides
- [ ] Nephrotic syndrome
- [ ] Henoch-Schonlein
- [ ] Acute vs chronic renal failure
- [ ] Urinary infection
- [ ] Transplantation and complications (cyclosporin A)
- [ ] Calculi
- [ ] Polycystic kidneys
- [ ] Renal tubular acidosis
- [ ] Papillary necrosis
- [ ] Other inherited disease (e.g. Alport's)
- [ ] List of causes of chronic renal failure

Investigation
- [ ] Concentrating mechanism
- [ ] Urinary electrolytes
- [ ] Microscopy/immunochemistry

Therapy
- [ ] Acid-base correction
- [ ] Steroids in GN
- [ ] Drugs and renal toxicity
- [ ] Site of diuretic action
- [ ] Renal osteodystrophy

NEUROLOGY

Basic science/physiology/anatomy
- [ ] Circle of Willis
- [ ] Brainstem
- [ ] Peripheral nerves
- [ ] Cranial nerves
- [ ] Autonomic nervous system

Clinical disorders/pathophysiology/complications
- [ ] Epilepsy
- [ ] Subarachnoid haemorrhage
- [ ] Dementia
- [ ] Transient global amnesia
- [ ] Motor neurone disease
- [ ] Brainstem vascular syndromes
- [ ] CVA
- [ ] Parkinsonism
- [ ] Other involuntary movements and tremor
- [ ] Dystrophia myotonica
- [ ] Myasthenia (and Eaton Lambert)
- [ ] Trigeminal neuralgia
- [ ] Benign intracranial hypertension
- [ ] Multiple sclerosis
- [ ] Prion diseases
- [ ] Tumours

Investigation
- [ ] CSF findings
- [ ] EEG/evoked potentials

Therapy
- [ ] Anti-epileptics
- [ ] Anti-Parkinsonian agents

PHARMACOLOGY

Basic science/physiology/anatomy
- [ ] Classification of drugs
- [ ] Mode of action
- [ ] Kinetics/disposition

- ☐ Enzyme induction
- ☐ Acetylator status
- ☐ Clinical trials

Clinical disorders/pathophysiology/complications
- ☐ Individual drugs
- ☐ Digoxin
- ☐ Monoamine oxidase inhibitors
- ☐ Anti-tuberculous drugs
- ☐ Anti-cancer chemotherapy
- ☐ Interactions (esp warfarin, phenytoin)
- ☐ Self poisoning and antidotes
- ☐ Renal excretion
- ☐ Hepatic metabolism
- ☐ Elderly patients
- ☐ Porphyria
- ☐ Side effects
- ☐ Drug induced lupus
- ☐ Photosensitivity
- ☐ Aplastic anaemia

Investigation
- ☐ Therapeutic monitoring

OPHTHALMOLOGY

- ☐ Causes of red eye
- ☐ Cataracts
- ☐ Papilloedema
- ☐ Visual field defects
- ☐ Central scotoma
- ☐ Enlarged blind spot

PSYCHIATRY

Basic science/physiology/anatomy
- ☐ Epidemiology
- ☐ Neurotransmitters
- ☐ Mental Health Act

Clinical disorders/pathophysiology/complications
- [ ] Schizophrenia (Schneiderian symptoms)
- [ ] Depression/bipolar affective illness
- [ ] Suicide/parasuicide
- [ ] Anorexia/bulimia
- [ ] Delirium/dementia
- [ ] Obsessional neurosis
- [ ] Alcohol dependency
- [ ] Organic brain disease
- [ ] Alzheimer's, Pick's, multi-infarct, CJD, etc

Investigation
- [ ] EEG in CJD
- [ ] Exclusion of organic disease

Therapy
- [ ] Antidepressants
- [ ] New SSRIs
- [ ] Lithium
- [ ] Delirium tremens

RESPIRATORY DISEASE

Basic science/physiology/anatomy
- [ ] Pulmonary anatomy
- [ ] Lateral CXR
- [ ] Blood gas analysis
- [ ] Oxygen dissociation curve
- [ ] Lung physiology

Clinical disorders/pathophysiology/complications
- [ ] Asthma
- [ ] Chronic bronchitis and emphysema
- [ ] Pleural effusion
- [ ] Bronchial carcinoma
- [ ] Allergic alveolitis
- [ ] Fibrosing alveolitis
- [ ] Acute respiratory failure
- [ ] Type 2 respiratory failure
- [ ] Upper lobe fibrosis
- [ ] Drug induced lung disease

- [ ] Cystic fibrosis
- [ ] Bronchiectasis
- [ ] Sarcoidosis
- [ ] Tuberculosis
- [ ] Mycoplasma
- [ ] Psittacosis
- [ ] Aspergillosis
- [ ] Pulmonary disease in AIDS
- [ ] Asbestos related lung disease
- [ ] Obstructive sleep apnoea
- [ ] Lung in SLE, polyarteritis, etc

Investigation
- [ ] Spirometry
- [ ] Transfer factor
- [ ] Lung volumes
- [ ] Flow-volume loop
- [ ] Compliance
- [ ] Bronchoalveolar lavage
- [ ] Cavitating lesion on CXR
- [ ] Calcification on CXR

Therapy
- [ ] Surgery for bronchial CA
- [ ] Asthma
- [ ] Pneumonia

RHEUMATOLOGY

Basic science/physiology/anatomy
- [ ] Autoantibodies

Clinical disorders/pathophysiology/complications
- [ ] Rheumatoid arthritis
- [ ] SLE
- [ ] Seronegative arthropathies
- [ ] Ankylosing spondylitis
- [ ] Gout/crystal arthritis
- [ ] Osteoarthritis
- [ ] Septic arthritis
- [ ] Paget's disease
- [ ] Endocrinology and arthropathy

- ☐ Extra-articular manifestations
- ☐ Viral arthritis
- ☐ Causes of kyphoscoliosis
- ☐ Behçet's disease
- ☐ Raynaud's phenomenon
- ☐ Reiter's syndrome

Investigation
- ☐ HLA typing
- ☐ Synovial fluid

Therapy
- ☐ Non-steroidal agents
- ☐ Second line agents
- ☐ Toxicity of drugs (esp penicillamine)

STATISTICS

- ☐ Clinical trials
- ☐ Chi squared
- ☐ Student's t test
- ☐ Correlation
- ☐ Parametric vs non-parametric
- ☐ Normal distribution
- ☐ Frequency distribution
- ☐ Skew distribution
- ☐ Mean, median, mode
- ☐ Standard deviation/variance/standard error
- ☐ Confidence intervals
- ☐ Probability (p value)
- ☐ Predictive value/type 1/ type 2 error

INSTRUCTIONS

In order to help MRCP Part 1 candidates revise for this difficult examination we have tried to follow as closely as possible the content and format of the official examination. Each question has an answer and teaching explanation which should provide a good basis for successful revision.

We suggest that you work on each set of 60 multiple choice questions as though it was a real examination. In other words, time yourself to spend no more than 2½ hours on each practice exam and do not obtain help from books, notes or other people while you are working. Plan to take this practice exam at a time when you will be undisturbed for a minimum of 2½ hours. Choose a well lit location free from distractions, keep your desk clear of other books or papers, have a clock or watch clearly visible. Equip yourself with a rubber and two well sharpened grade B pencils.

As you work through each question in this book be sure to mark a tick ('True') or a cross ('False') in the answer boxes next to each question. If you need to indicate 'Don't Know', then leave the answer space blank. Thus when you have completed the paper you can mark your own answers against the answers and explanations given at the end of the book. Do not be tempted to look at the questions before sitting down to take each test as it will not then represent a valid mock exam.

When you have finished the exam, go through your answers to make sure that you have not made any mistakes. Do not feel that you have to spend the full 2½ hours available reconsidering your answers if you are confident about your work. Give yourself one mark for a correct answer and deduct a mark for an incorrect answer. Answers left blank score zero. Highlight the questions that you got wrong in the book. Using the analysis of subject areas in the exams, which is given in at the back of the book, will help you concentrate your limited revision time on the subjects that need it most.

Royal Colleges of Physicians

SURNAME

INITIALS

EXAMINATION NO.

(0)	(0)	(0)	(0)
(1)	(1)	(1)	(1)
(2)	(2)	(2)	(2)
(3)	(3)	(3)	(3)
(4)	(4)	(4)	(4)
(5)	(5)	(5)	(5)
(6)	(6)	(6)	(6)
(7)	(7)	(7)	(7)
(8)	(8)	(8)	(8)
(9)	(9)	(9)	(9)

Please use 2B PENCIL only. Rub out all errors thoroughly.
Mark rectangles like ━ **NOT like this** ∕ ∦ ✗

T ▭ = **TRUE**   F ▭ = **FALSE**   DK ▭ = **DON'T KNOW**

	A	B	C	D	E			A	B	C	D	E
1	T F DK	T F DK	T F DK	T F DK	T F DK		**16**	T F DK	T F DK	T F DK	T F DK	T F DK
2	T F DK	T F DK	T F DK	T F DK	T F DK		**17**	T F DK	T F DK	T F DK	T F DK	T F DK
3	T F DK	T F DK	T F DK	T F DK	T F DK		**18**	T F DK	T F DK	T F DK	T F DK	T F DK
4	T F DK	T F DK	T F DK	T F DK	T F DK		**19**	T F DK	T F DK	T F DK	T F DK	T F DK
5	T F DK	T F DK	T F DK	T F DK	T F DK		**20**	T F DK	T F DK	T F DK	T F DK	T F DK
6	T F DK	T F DK	T F DK	T F DK	T F DK		**21**	T F DK	T F DK	T F DK	T F DK	T F DK
7	T F DK	T F DK	T F DK	T F DK	T F DK		**22**	T F DK	T F DK	T F DK	T F DK	T F DK
8	T F DK	T F DK	T F DK	T F DK	T F DK		**23**	T F DK	T F DK	T F DK	T F DK	T F DK
9	T F DK	T F DK	T F DK	T F DK	T F DK		**24**	T F DK	T F DK	T F DK	T F DK	T F DK
10	T F DK	T F DK	T F DK	T F DK	T F DK		**25**	T F DK	T F DK	T F DK	T F DK	T F DK
11	T F DK	T F DK	T F DK	T F DK	T F DK		**26**	T F DK	T F DK	T F DK	T F DK	T F DK
12	T F DK	T F DK	T F DK	T F DK	T F DK		**27**	T F DK	T F DK	T F DK	T F DK	T F DK
13	T F DK	T F DK	T F DK	T F DK	T F DK		**28**	T F DK	T F DK	T F DK	T F DK	T F DK
14	T F DK	T F DK	T F DK	T F DK	T F DK		**29**	T F DK	T F DK	T F DK	T F DK	T F DK
15	T F DK	T F DK	T F DK	T F DK	T F DK		**30**	T F DK	T F DK	T F DK	T F DK	T F DK

60 questions: Time allowed 2½ hours.
Mark your answers with a tick (True) or a cross (False) in the box provided.
Leave the box blank for 'Don't know'.

1   Proto-oncogenes

☐   A   are carcinogenic retroviruses
☐   B   are only expressed in malignant tissues
☐   C   control cell growth and differentiation
☐   D   are transiently upregulated by growth factors
☐   E   inactivate oncogenes

2   The diastolic blood pressure readings of 1000 8-year-old children were found to have a statistically normal distribution with a mean value of 61 mm Hg and a standard deviation of 8 mm Hg:

☐   A   the mean and standard deviation completely define the distribution of diastolic blood pressures for this age group
☐   B   the mean diastolic blood pressure for this sample is equal to that for the whole population
☐   C   95% of the sample data lie within an interval defined by the mean ± 2 standard deviations (i.e. the range 45–77 mm Hg)
☐   D   the median is 53 (i.e. 1 standard deviation below the mean)
☐   E   the variance is 64 (i.e. the square of the standard deviation)

3   The following occur in anorexia nervosa:

☐   A   amenorrhoea
☐   B   osteoporosis
☐   C   hyperkalaemia
☐   D   raised plasma cortisol
☐   E   depressed mood

4   The following are autosomal dominant:

☐   A   Wilson's disease
☐   B   arachnodactyly
☐   C   familial polyposis coli
☐   D   tuberous sclerosis
☐   E   limb girdle muscular dystrophy (Erb's)

1

5   Characteristic features of HIV seroconversion illness include

☐   A   oral ulceration
☐   B   petechial rash
☐   C   positive HIV P24 antigen
☐   D   aseptic meningitis
☐   E   an association with good prognosis

6   A radial nerve lesion above the elbow leads to

☐   A   weakness of brachialis
☐   B   weakness of abductor pollicis longus
☐   C   weakness of extensor pollicis brevis
☐   D   weakness of first lumbrical
☐   E   sensory loss affecting skin over medial aspect of dorsal hand
           surface

7   Multiple seborrhoeic warts

☐   A   are most commonly found on the limbs
☐   B   are usually infective
☐   C   are best removed by excision
☐   D   have a recognized association with internal malignancy
☐   E   are a feature of Cowden's disease

8   The following are true of tuberculosis in the UK:

☐   A   HIV-positive individuals should not receive BCG
☐   B   it occurs in less than 5% of contacts
☐   C   sputum-positive patients are non-infectious after 2 weeks of
           therapy
☐   D   drug resistance is now greater than 10%
☐   E   large pleural effusions require steroid therapy

9   In myasthenia gravis

☐   A   antibodies to acetylcholine receptors are present
☐   B   antibodies to smooth muscle are associated with the presence of a thymoma
☐   C   tendon reflexes are usually absent
☐   D   pupillary reflexes are abnormal
☐   E   large doses of anticholinesterases may precipitate weakness

10   A cardiac murmur is likely to be innocent (i.e. not associated with demonstrable structural abnormality) if

☐   A   it is diastolic
☐   B   the only finding is a soft ejection systolic murmur at the left sternal edge in a healthy young child
☐   C   it is associated with a palpable thrill
☐   D   it is systolic with an ejection click
☐   E   it is continuous, and disappears on neck vein compression or when lying down

11   Hepatitis B virus

☐   A   e antigen is a cleavage product of core antigen
☐   B   is an RNA virus
☐   C   replication is inhibited by interferon
☐   D   is required for hepatitis D infection
☐   E   binds to hepatocytes via e antigen

12   In untreated 21 hydroxylase deficiency

☐   A   female clitoromegaly is characteristic
☐   B   pregnanetriol excretion is increased
☐   C   plasma renin activity is suppressed
☐   D   serum progesterone level is reduced
☐   E   delayed puberty is common in affected males

13 Intestinal pseudo-obstruction may be a manifestation of

☐ A amyloidosis
☐ B squamous cell carcinoma of the lung
☐ C lead poisoning
☐ D Parkinson's disease
☐ E sarcoidosis

14 The cause of thrombocytopenia in the following conditions is correctly assigned in each case:

☐ A acute leukaemia: marrow aplasia
☐ B systemic lupus erythematosus: platelet antibodies
☐ C Gram-negative septicaemia: marrow aplasia
☐ D massive transfusion: platelet antibodies
☐ E splenomegaly from any cause: sequestration

15 Pericarditis is commonly associated with

☐ A rheumatoid arthritis
☐ B scleroderma
☐ C mixed connective tissue disease
☐ D Reiter's disease
☐ E Still's disease

16 A diagnosis of diabetes mellitus is confirmed by the presence of

☐ A generalized pruritus
☐ B fasting venous plasma glucose 6.8 mmol/l
☐ C glycosuria
☐ D polyuria and polydipsia
☐ E venous plasma glucose 11.2 mmol/l, 2 hours after 75 g oral glucose

17 Thrombosis of the posterior inferior cerebellar artery causes

- ☐ A infarction of the medial medulla oblongata
- ☐ B contralateral partial ptosis
- ☐ C ipsilateral loss of pain and temperature sensation in the limbs
- ☐ D diplopia
- ☐ E contralateral hemiplegia

18 In patients with rheumatic fever the following indicate carditis:

- ☐ A pericarditis
- ☐ B diastolic murmur
- ☐ C prolonged PR interval
- ☐ D sinus arrhythmia
- ☐ E cardiomegaly

19 The following drugs have been associated with impairment of glucose tolerance:

- ☐ A bendrofluazide
- ☐ B combined oestrogen/progestogen oral contraceptive pill
- ☐ C glipizide
- ☐ D prednisolone
- ☐ E spironolactone

20 Ciprofloxacin has good activity against

- ☐ A *Mycobacterium tuberculosis*
- ☐ B *Salmonella paratyphi*
- ☐ C *Streptococcus pneumoniae*
- ☐ D *Legionella pneumophila*
- ☐ E *Bacteroides fragilis*

21 In autoimmune thyroid eye disease

- ☐ A exophthalmos is due to retro-orbital fluid
- ☐ B there is exacerbation by cigarette smoking
- ☐ C diplopia is normally due to 3rd nerve palsy
- ☐ D high dose steroids are mandatory
- ☐ E improvement follows 131-Iodine treatment

22 The following suggest a diagnosis of gluten sensitivity:

- ☐ A Howell-Jolly bodies in the peripheral blood
- ☐ B a positive C14 breath test
- ☐ C aphthous ulceration of the mouth
- ☐ D osteoporosis
- ☐ E focal biliary cirrhosis

23 Anaphylaxis

- ☐ A involves mast cells and basophils
- ☐ B is triggered by binding of monomeric IgE alone
- ☐ C is manifest by vasoconstriction
- ☐ D can be caused by administration of antibody
- ☐ E is an example of a type 1 reaction

24 Apoprotein A1

- ☐ A is directly related to risk of ischaemic heart disease
- ☐ B levels are increased in nephrotic syndrome
- ☐ C is associated with high density lipoprotein
- ☐ D is a component of chylomicrons
- ☐ E has beta mobility on an electrophoretic strip

25 The following are true of membranous glomerulonephritis:

- [ ] A immune-complex mediated aetiology
- [ ] B 35% chance of progression to renal failure
- [ ] C strong association with Hodgkin's disease
- [ ] D the disease does not recur in renal allografts
- [ ] E it is a common renal lesion in patients with rheumatoid arthritis

26 In sleep disturbance the following statements are valid:

- [ ] A 55% of insomnias are secondary
- [ ] B alcohol increases total sleep time
- [ ] C benzodiazepines may cause akathisia
- [ ] D narcolepsy usually presents in the first to second decade
- [ ] E patients with hypersomnia have an irresistible urge to sleep

27 Pulmonary nodules are found in

- [ ] A rheumatoid arthritis
- [ ] B systemic sclerosis
- [ ] C systemic lupus erythematosus
- [ ] D Wegener's granulomatosis
- [ ] E polyarteritis nodosa

28 The following statements are true of Huntington's disease (chorea):

- [ ] A the gene is localized on the short arm of chromosome 5
- [ ] B it is associated with a cortical dementia
- [ ] C prominent rigidity with little chorea is associated with a juvenile onset
- [ ] D the prominent abnormality on CT imaging is atrophy of the caudate nucleus
- [ ] E L-dopa medication typically improves chorea

29 Haemarthrosis is seen in

☐ A haemophilia B
☐ B sickle cell disease
☐ C Charcot joints
☐ D thrombocytopenia
☐ E pyrophosphate arthritis

30 Hyperprolactinaemia is a recognized feature of

☐ A thyrotoxicosis
☐ B acromegaly
☐ C treatment with clozapine
☐ D pseudoseizures
☐ E hypothyroidism

31 The risk of atheromatous coronary disease is increased

☐ A in WHO type 1 hyperlipidaemia
☐ B when HDL cholesterol >2.0 mmol/l
☐ C when proteinuria complicates type 2 diabetes
☐ D in heterozygous familial hypercholesterolaemia
☐ E when LDL cholesterol >4.5 mmol/l

32 Diffuse oesophageal spasm is characterized by

☐ A central chest pain relieved by glyceryl trinitrate
☐ B effort related pain
☐ C the presence of a corkscrew oesophagus on barium swallow
☐ D the absence of simultaneous contractions on manometry
☐ E a low incidence below the age of 50

33 A lesion of the third cranial nerve causes

☐ A an afferent pupillary defect
☐ B a divergent strabismus
☐ C inability to adduct the affected eye
☐ D contralateral hemiplegia
☐ E miosis

34 Features of cardiac syncope include

☐ A transient unconsciousness with rapid return to consciousness
☐ B preceding aura
☐ C distinction from epilepsy by absence of tonic/clonic phases
☐ D tachyarrhythmias
☐ E occurrence in the erect or supine position

35 Rabies virus

☐ A transmission may be reduced by washing bite wounds
☐ B infection is diagnosed by positive serology during the incubation period
☐ C infection survival has improved with modern intensive care
☐ D infection may be diagnosed by skin punch biopsy from the neck
☐ E post-exposure prophylaxis is by simultaneous active and passive immunisation

36 Neurofibromatosis is associated with

☐ A phaeochromocytoma
☐ B retinal phacoma
☐ C acoustic neuroma
☐ D meningioma
☐ E plexiform neuroma

37 Specific precipitating antibodies are present in

- ☐ A byssinosis
- ☐ B bagassosis
- ☐ C histoplasmosis
- ☐ D fibrosing alveolitis
- ☐ E bird fancier's lung

38 Iron deficiency

- ☐ A is associated with a reduction in the serum transferrin concentration
- ☐ B results in defective globin synthesis
- ☐ C can result in gastrointestinal malabsorption
- ☐ D is seen in patients with paroxysmal nocturnal haemoglobinuria
- ☐ E is associated with glossitis

39 Recognized features of hypothermia include

- ☐ A pancreatitis
- ☐ B left shift of the haemoglobin-oxygen dissociation curve
- ☐ C myotonia
- ☐ D impaired shivering thermogenesis
- ☐ E acute hepatic necrosis

40 Tetracycline

- ☐ A is contraindicated in renal failure
- ☐ B may cause staining of developing bones and teeth
- ☐ C is the drug of first choice for *Legionella pneumophila* infections
- ☐ D is effective in Rickettsial infections
- ☐ E is useful in the treatment of gonococcal urethritis

41 Anaemia in chronic renal failure

☐ A becomes evident when glomerular filtration rate falls below
      30 ml/min
☐ B is reversed by dialysis
☐ C is least marked in patients with polycystic kidneys
☐ D is tolerated by most patients because of an increase in red cell 2,3
      diphosphoglycerate (2,3 DPG)
☐ E due to iron deficiency is recognized by a low serum iron

42 Insulin resistance

☐ A is associated with raised HDL-cholesterol
☐ B is associated with hypertension
☐ C is unaffected by physical training
☐ D is characterized clinically by acanthosis nigricans
☐ E is due to a reduced number of insulin receptors

**43 An increase in plasma digoxin levels would be expected on
introduction of**

☐ A amiodarone
☐ B nifedipine
☐ C quinidine
☐ D cholestyramine
☐ E rifampicin

**44 The bioavailability of the following drugs is increased in the
presence of hepatic cirrhosis:**

☐ A digoxin
☐ B propranolol
☐ C metoclopramide
☐ D gentamicin
☐ E imipramine

45 Features of acromegaly include

- ☐ A carpal tunnel syndrome
- ☐ B elevated serum IGF-1 concentration
- ☐ C tunnel vision
- ☐ D increased risk of colonic carcinoma
- ☐ E frontal sinus destruction

46 Chronic myeloid leukaemia

- ☐ A is associated with a raised serum vitamin B12 level
- ☐ B can evolve into both acute myeloid or acute lymphoid leukaemia
- ☐ C commonly presents with lymphadenopathy and massive splenomegaly
- ☐ D is associated with translocation between chromosomes 8 and 22
- ☐ E can be effectively treated by alpha-interferon

47 The following helminths may cause respiratory symptoms:

- ☐ A *Ascaris lumbricoides*
- ☐ B *Necator americanus*
- ☐ C *Paragonimus westermani*
- ☐ D *Strongyloides stercoralis*
- ☐ E *Ancylostoma braziliensis*

48 Osteopenia is associated with

- ☐ A early menopause
- ☐ B cigarette smoking
- ☐ C reflex sympathetic dystrophy
- ☐ D testosterone deficiency
- ☐ E precocious puberty

49 In the leg

- ☐ A spasticity in a patient with hemiplegia is most pronounced in the extensor muscles
- ☐ B weakness in a patient with hemiplegia is most pronounced in the flexor muscles
- ☐ C sensory loss affecting skin over the lateral aspect of the lower leg may be due to a femoral nerve palsy
- ☐ D weakness of knee extension may be due to a sciatic nerve palsy
- ☐ E foot drop may be due to a common peroneal nerve palsy

50 In obstructive sleep apnoea

- ☐ A obesity is an important factor
- ☐ B onset before middle age is usual
- ☐ C insomnia is the main complaint
- ☐ D polycythaemia may be present
- ☐ E sedatives should be avoided

51 The following adverse effects are associated with the use of enalapril:

- ☐ A angioneurotic oedema
- ☐ B cough in around 10% of patients
- ☐ C retroperitoneal fibrosis
- ☐ D acute renal failure
- ☐ E hypercholesterolaemia

52 Complications seen in patients suffering from sickle cell disease include

- ☐ A priapism
- ☐ B pneumothorax
- ☐ C cataracts
- ☐ D renal papillary necrosis
- ☐ E hyposplenism

53 The following are typical clinical features of Parkinson's disease:

☐ A pseudobulbar palsy
☐ B hypophonia
☐ C supranuclear gaze palsy
☐ D intention tremor
☐ E rigidity

54 The following dusts are highly fibrogenic to the lung:

☐ A silica
☐ B iron oxide
☐ C tungsten carbide
☐ D aluminium
☐ E tin

55 Tall R waves in ECG lead V1 are seen in

☐ A posterior myocardial infarction
☐ B acute pulmonary embolism
☐ C right bundle branch block
☐ D uncomplicated tricuspid atresia
☐ E Wolff-Parkinson-White syndrome

56 Ulcerative colitis is classically characterized by

☐ A fistula formation
☐ B diarrhoea
☐ C cobblestoning of mucosa
☐ D pseudopolyps
☐ E rectal involvement

57 The classical rash of typhoid fever (rose spots)

☐ A is a poor prognostic sign
☐ B begins on the extremities
☐ C is petechial
☐ D does not occur in paratyphoid
☐ E usually lasts a week or more

58 In the management of acute myocardial infarction, intravenous streptokinase

☐ A reduces mortality by 50% if given within 12 hours
☐ B is more effective than alteplase for anterior infarcts
☐ C shortens the partial thromboplastin time
☐ D efficacy is enhanced by recent streptococcal infection
☐ E is contraindicated by systolic BP >200 mm Hg

59 The following are autosomal recessively inherited conditions:

☐ A Alport's syndrome
☐ B cystinosis
☐ C cystinuria
☐ D nephrogenic diabetes insipidus
☐ E primary hyperoxaluria

60 The following statements apply to bronchial carcinoma:

☐ A screening is of little benefit
☐ B it is more common in urban areas
☐ C nickel is a recognized risk factor
☐ D the incidence in females is rising
☐ E haemoptysis suggests a poor prognosis

END OF EXAM 1

Go over your answers until your time is up. Answers and teaching notes are on page 77.

60 questions: Time allowed 2½ hours.
Mark your answers with a tick (True) or a cross (False) in the box provided.
Leave the box blank for 'Don't know'.

1 Hepatocellular carcinoma

- ☐ A is more common in women
- ☐ B is usually associated with chronic hepatitis B
- ☐ C may present as an acute abdomen
- ☐ D needs a liver biopsy to confirm the diagnosis
- ☐ E rarely produces hepatomegaly

2 Disseminated intravascular coagulation

- ☐ A is often characterized by neurological presentation
- ☐ B produces fragmented red cells
- ☐ C produces thrombocytopenia
- ☐ D responds to heparin therapy in the majority of cases
- ☐ E is characterised by raised fibrin degradation products

3 Scleritis is seen in

- ☐ A rheumatoid arthritis
- ☐ B SLE
- ☐ C Wegener's granulomatosis
- ☐ D ankylosing spondylitis
- ☐ E giant cell arteritis

4 Predisposing factors for diabetic neuropathic ulceration include

- ☐ A motor neuropathy
- ☐ B metformin treatment
- ☐ C normal sympathetic nerve function
- ☐ D simple background retinopathy
- ☐ E skin callus

5   The following features typically occur in complex partial seizures of temporal lobe onset:

- ☐   A   aura of fear accompanied by an epigastric sensation
- ☐   B   primitive visual aura
- ☐   C   jamais vu phenomenon
- ☐   D   automatisms
- ☐   E   versive seizures

6   In congestive cardiomyopathy the following features may be found:

- ☐   A   protodiastolic gallop
- ☐   B   clinical improvement following intramuscular thiamine
- ☐   C   mural thrombus formation
- ☐   D   a tendency to ventricular arrhythmias
- ☐   E   angiotensin converting enzyme inhibitors may improve symptoms and survival

7   The following drugs may cause impairment of renal function:

- ☐   A   captopril
- ☐   B   verapamil
- ☐   C   glyceryl trinitrate
- ☐   D   gentamicin
- ☐   E   indomethacin

8   Pneumococcal vaccination should be given to patients

- ☐   A   who are HIV positive
- ☐   B   who are heterozygous for Hb S
- ☐   C   who have had a splenectomy
- ☐   D   every five years where indicated
- ☐   E   prior to travel to countries with high rates of penicillin-resistant pneumococci

9   Total serum thyroxine levels are reduced by

☐ A   pregnancy
☐ B   phenytoin treatment
☐ C   panhypopituitarism
☐ D   combined oral contraceptives
☐ E   salicylate

10   Gallstones are associated with

☐ A   Gilbert's syndrome
☐ B   Crohn's disease
☐ C   familial hypercholesterolaemia
☐ D   hereditary spherocytosis
☐ E   cystic fibrosis

11   Complement deficiency

☐ A   is described for all 11 classical pathway proteins
☐ B   affecting C1 esterase inhibitor leads to angio-oedema
☐ C   heterozygotes have half normal levels, and homozygotes have no
         active proteins
☐ D   genes are located in the MHC region
☐ E   affecting C2 may be associated with connective tissue disease

12   Tumour necrosis factor

☐ A   causes cachexia
☐ B   is produced by bronchogenic carcinoma
☐ C   enhances insulin sensitivity
☐ D   is elevated in septic shock
☐ E   circulates bound to alpha-2 macroglobulin

13 The following are recognized complications in dialysis patients:

☐ A carpal tunnel syndrome
☐ B encephalopathy
☐ C cardiac arrest
☐ D high incidence of cardiovascular disease
☐ E skin tumours

14 The following are true of anxiety states:

☐ A chest pain may be a presenting symptom
☐ B may present with persistent memory impairment
☐ C difficulty in exhaling is common
☐ D low mood and early morning wakening are invariably present
☐ E sweating is common

15 Recognized findings in a Pancoast tumour are

☐ A erosion of the first rib
☐ B ipsilateral Horner's syndrome
☐ C paralysis of muscles in the arm
☐ D pain in the arm radiating to the 4th and 5th fingers
☐ E gangrene of the fingers on the same side

16 Myotonia

☐ A is typically exacerbated by exercise
☐ B occurs in hyperkalaemic periodic paralysis
☐ C and muscle hypertrophy may be associated
☐ D may be associated with cataracts
☐ E produces characteristic EMG findings

17 Features of psychogenic pain include

- ☐ A muscular tension
- ☐ B good response to analgesics
- ☐ C benefit from antidepressants
- ☐ D inconsistency with anatomical patterns of innervation
- ☐ E a prolonged course of unusual severity

18 Actions of glucagon include

- ☐ A stimulation of hepatic glycogenolysis
- ☐ B inhibition of insulin secretion
- ☐ C stimulation of hepatic gluconeogenesis
- ☐ D inhibition of adenyl cyclase
- ☐ E a positive cardiac inotropic effect

19 Drugs which lower serum LDL cholesterol concentration include

- ☐ A simvastatin
- ☐ B cholestyramine
- ☐ C propranolol
- ☐ D fenofibrate
- ☐ E omega-3 marine oil

20 The long acting somatostatin analogue octreotide

- ☐ A decreases small intestinal transit time
- ☐ B produces marked dilatation of portal veins
- ☐ C can only be given intravenously
- ☐ D stimulates pancreatic exocrine secretion
- ☐ E reduces splanchnic arterial blood flow

21 The posterior interosseous nerve

☐ A is a branch of the median nerve
☐ B supplies brachioradialis
☐ C supplies supinator
☐ D supplies flexor pollicis longus
☐ E supplies opponens pollicis

22 The following are associated with increased likelihood of stroke:

☐ A mitral annular calcification
☐ B atrial fibrillation in non-rheumatic heart disease
☐ C atrial fibrillation in rheumatic heart disease
☐ D coarctation of the aorta
☐ E patent foramen ovale

23 Mumps virus infection

☐ A is asymptomatic in 40%
☐ B with raised amylase is diagnostic of pancreatitis
☐ C is complicated by meningitis in less than 1% of cases
☐ D is due to an RNA virus
☐ E is a recognized cause of oophoritis

24 In multiple sclerosis, plaques of demyelination characteristically occur in

☐ A cerebral cortex
☐ B subcortical white matter
☐ C optic nerves
☐ D anterior horn cells
☐ E cervical cord

25 In bronchoalveolar lavage

- ☐ A normally 90% of cells are macrophages
- ☐ B extrinsic allergic alveolitis typically produces a high neutrophil percentage
- ☐ C sarcoid causes an increase in T4-lymphocytes
- ☐ D alveolar proteinosis may produce a diagnostic appearance
- ☐ E smokers have a higher neutrophil percentage than normals

26 A normochromic-normocytic anaemia can be seen in the following circumstances

- ☐ A hypopituitarism
- ☐ B sideroblastic anaemia
- ☐ C acute blood loss
- ☐ D aplastic anaemia
- ☐ E long-term phenytoin administration

27 Correct associations of tumours and circulating markers include

- ☐ A ovarian carcinoma and CA125
- ☐ B hepatoma and human chorionic gonadotrophin
- ☐ C teratoma and alpha fetoprotein
- ☐ D medullary thyroid carcinoma and thyroglobulin
- ☐ E osteosarcoma and PTH-related peptide

28 Metoclopramide

- ☐ A is effective as a hypoglycaemic agent
- ☐ B delays gastric emptying time
- ☐ C acts centrally as a dopamine agonist
- ☐ D causes extrapyramidal reactions in young women
- ☐ E may cause galactorrhoea

29 Renal failure in multiple myeloma is associated with

☐ A amyloidosis
☐ B hyperuricaemia
☐ C intravenous pyelography
☐ D glomerular destruction by precipitation of kappa and lambda light chains in Bowman's space
☐ E hypercalcaemia

30 p53

☐ A suppresses cell division
☐ B is a viral protein
☐ C mutation promotes tumorigenesis
☐ D controls normal development
☐ E is required for apoptosis

31 Concerning calcium channel blockers:

☐ A they inhibit slow calcium efflux during stage 2 of the cardiac action potential
☐ B diltiazem increases AV nodal refractoriness
☐ C nifedipine is safe in pregnancy
☐ D i.v. verapamil can safely be given to patients in ventricular tachycardia
☐ E gum hypertrophy is a side-effect of the dihydropyridines

32 Enzyme induction

☐ A with anticonvulsants may cause osteomalacia
☐ B contributes to tolerance to the effects of atenolol
☐ C can cause failure of the contraceptive pill
☐ D may occur as a result of smoking
☐ E lowers plasma bilirubin concentration

33 Klinefelter's syndrome leads to

- ☐ A infertility
- ☐ B gynaecomastia
- ☐ C mental retardation
- ☐ D high serum gonadotrophins
- ☐ E premature balding

34 Warm-type autoimmune haemolytic anaemia (AIHA)

- ☐ A is a recognized complication of acute lymphoblastic leukaemia
- ☐ B is rarely mediated by IgG immunoglobulins
- ☐ C occurs following infection with *Mycoplasma pneumoniae*
- ☐ D is usually associated with a positive Coombs test
- ☐ E is recognized following administration of L-dopa

35 *Schistosoma mansoni* infection

- ☐ A is common in the Indian subcontinent
- ☐ B may present with spastic paraparesis
- ☐ C does not cause cercarial dermatitis
- ☐ D predisposes to recurrent salmonella bacteraemia
- ☐ E is treated with praziquantel

36 Hypomagnesaemia is a feature of

- ☐ A diabetic ketoacidosis
- ☐ B chronic diarrhoea
- ☐ C loop diuretic toxicity
- ☐ D acute myocardial infarction
- ☐ E primary hyperparathyroidism

37 Significant negative inotropic action is a feature of

- [ ] A diltiazem
- [ ] B lisinopril
- [ ] C propafenone
- [ ] D bisoprolol
- [ ] E thyroxine

38 The following are causally related:

- [ ] A melphalan and pulmonary fibrosis
- [ ] B hydrochlorothiazide and pulmonary oedema
- [ ] C barbiturates and hyperventilation
- [ ] D phenytoin and SLE
- [ ] E prostaglandin F2 alpha and bronchodilatation

39 Parkinson-like extrapyramidal effects occur during treatment with

- [ ] A haloperidol
- [ ] B imipramine
- [ ] C prochlorperazine
- [ ] D phenytoin
- [ ] E trifluoperazine

40 Multiple myeloma

- [ ] A occasionally occurs in the absence of a serum paraprotein
- [ ] B is a cause of a leucoerythroblastic blood picture
- [ ] C presents with bone pain in a minority of cases
- [ ] D is a recognized cause of carpal tunnel syndrome
- [ ] E has a peak incidence in the 5th decade

41   In the upper gastrointestinal tract

☐   A   ranitidine competitively blocks histamine H1 receptors
☐   B   cisapride has anticholinergic actions
☐   C   omeprazole lowers intragastric pH
☐   D   domperidone stimulates dopamine D2 receptors
☐   E   sucralfate is a potent acid neutralising agent

42   In acute asthma

☐   A   hydrocortisone is frequently required
☐   B   antibiotics should normally be given
☐   C   sedatives may be useful
☐   D   high flow oxygen therapy is usually indicated
☐   E   a high pCO_2 is of little consequence

43   In Addisonian pernicious anaemia (PA)

☐   A   the serum folate is often raised in association with a low red cell folate
☐   B   antibodies to intrinsic factor are found in the serum of 90% of patients
☐   C   a response to treatment with corticosteroids is common
☐   D   is associated with a higher than normal incidence of carcinoma of the stomach
☐   E   infertility is a rare presentation

44   A third heart sound in a 45-year-old man

☐   A   is a sign of heart disease
☐   B   excludes significant A-V valve stenosis
☐   C   could be due to tricuspid regurgitation
☐   D   is a feature of constrictive pericarditis
☐   E   could indicate hypertensive heart disease

45 The following statements are true of Creutzfeldt-Jakob disease:

☐ A it is slowly progressive over many years
☐ B myoclonus is an early clinical feature
☐ C EEG is usually normal
☐ D it is associated with a spongiform histological change in the brain
☐ E approximately 10% of cases are familial

46 The membrane attack complex of the complement system is

☐ A formed by alternative pathway activation
☐ B deficient in paroxysmal nocturnal haemoglobinuria
☐ C inhibited by VLDL
☐ D only active against heterologous cells
☐ E responsible for hereditary angioneurotic oedema

47 The following statements concerning asbestosis are true:

☐ A it occurs only after heavy occupational exposure
☐ B pleural plaques are pre-malignant
☐ C carcinoma of the bronchus is a recognized complication
☐ D it is frequently associated with positive anti-nuclear factor
☐ E it produces pulmonary nodules as well as marked fibrosis

48 The following statements are true of Normal Pressure Hydrocephalus (NPH):

☐ A it causes a cortical dementia
☐ B spasticity in the lower limbs is greater than that in the upper limbs
☐ C urinary incontinence is a late clinical manifestation
☐ D structural imaging (CT and MRI) reveals 'slit-like' lateral ventricles
☐ E clinical improvement may follow a CSF shunting procedure

49 HLA molecules

- ☐ A are encoded for by genes on chromosome 6
- ☐ B are constitutively expressed only on leucocytes
- ☐ C form part of the T cell receptor
- ☐ D present antigen
- ☐ E are associated with beta-2 microglobulin

50 The time taken to walk 10 metres was recorded in 50 patients who had suffered a stroke. The observations were found to be distributed symmetrically about the mean (47 seconds).

- ☐ A the observations, being symmetrical about the mean, must follow a Normal distribution
- ☐ B if the observations had been found to be positively skewed, their mode would have been less than the mean
- ☐ C the median time to walk 10 metres is equal to the 50th percentile
- ☐ D computing the variance of the observations would provide a measure of their spread about the mean
- ☐ E computing the standard deviation of the observations would provide a measure of the reliability of the mean

51 Common features of bulimia nervosa include

- ☐ A low body weight
- ☐ B recurrent episodes of binge eating
- ☐ C distorted body image
- ☐ D self induced vomiting
- ☐ E laxative abuse

52 An X-chromosome containing an abnormal gene is found in the following:

- ☐ A haemophilia B
- ☐ B Duchenne muscular dystrophy
- ☐ C congenital pyloric stenosis
- ☐ D nephrogenic diabetes insipidus
- ☐ E ataxia telangiectasia

53 In HIV-positive patients, prophylactic agents are of proven benefit in reducing the incidence of the following opportunistic infections:

☐ A cytomegalovirus (CMV) retinitis
☐ B pneumocystic carinii pneumonia (PCP)
☐ C mycobacterium avium complex bacteraemia (MACBAC)
☐ D toxoplasma encephalitis
☐ E cryptosporidial diarrhoea

54 The following statements are true:

☐ A the ulnar nerve supplies the first and second lumbricals
☐ B the ulnar nerve supplies the majority of the intrinsic muscles of the hand
☐ C the median nerve supplies flexor carpi radialis
☐ D the radial nerve supplies the dorsal interossei
☐ E the radial nerve supplies adductor pollicis

55 Alopecia areata

☐ A is a scarring process with permanent loss of follicles
☐ B is associated with autoimmune thyroid disease
☐ C is confined to scalp hairs
☐ D is a recognized association of Down's syndrome
☐ E may be associated with nail changes

56 In community acquired pneumonia

☐ A the most common causative organism is *S. pneumoniae*
☐ B mycoplasma occurs in five yearly epidemics
☐ C a definite pathogen is unusual
☐ D serum urea greater than 7 mmol/l is a bad prognostic sign
☐ E type II respiratory failure is common

57 In motor neurone disease

☐ A sphincters are involved late in the disease
☐ B there may be associated dementia
☐ C root pain is common
☐ D the extraocular muscles are spared
☐ E familial cases are described

58 Mitral stenosis

☐ A is more common in women than in men
☐ B is of rheumatic aetiology in approximately 50% of cases
☐ C is characterized by shortness of breath on effort
☐ D is associated with tricuspid regurgitation usually due to rheumatic involvement of the tricuspid valve
☐ E is excluded if the patient is in sinus rhythm

59 Cystic fibrosis

☐ A affects 1 in every 1000 infants
☐ B is due to a specific mutation of the cystic fibrosis transmembrane conductance regulator gene
☐ C cystic fibrosis conductance regulator gene therapy is delivered by a viral vector
☐ D is due to defective $Na^+:K^+$ transport
☐ E gene therapy need only be given once

60 Polycystic ovary syndrome

☐ A occurs in 20% of young women
☐ B causes anovulatory infertility
☐ C leads to elevated serum FSH levels
☐ D is associated with hyperprolactinaemia
☐ E is common in ballet dancers

END OF EXAM 2

Go over your answers until your time is up. Answers and teaching notes are on page 89.

60 questions: Time allowed 2½ hours.
Mark your answers with a tick (True) or a cross (False) in the box provided.
Leave the box blank for 'Don't know'.

1   Concerning anti-nuclear factors:

☐ A   antibodies to ds-DNA are highly specific for SLE
☐ B   they may be detected by use of a haemoflagellate
☐ C   anti ss-DNA occurs in 90% of SLE patients
☐ D   immunofluorescence staining is of great diagnostic value
☐ E   titres reliably reflect disease activity

2   Anti-phospholipid antibodies

☐ A   prolong the bleeding time
☐ B   are associated with recurrent spontaneous abortion
☐ C   have a high positive predictive value for SLE
☐ D   occur in culture negative endocarditis
☐ E   are associated with Addison's disease

3   The following are true of urinary infection in adults:

☐ A   *Proteus mirabilis* is the most common offending organism in
        general practice
☐ B   renal damage by analgesics is a predisposing factor
☐ C   bladder neck obstruction predisposes to infection
☐ D   bacterial colonisation of bladder urine is usually due to descending
        infection from the kidney
☐ E   chronic renal failure is a common feature

4   In obsessive–compulsive disorder

☐ A   obsessional thought is recognised by the patient as being his own
☐ B   women are more commonly affected than men
☐ C   obsessional thoughts are usually pleasant in nature
☐ D   depression is unusual
☐ E   two-thirds of cases have improved at the end of one year

5   Pulmonary abscess formation secondary to aspiration is characteristically seen in

- ☐   A   basal segments of the lower lobes
- ☐   B   apical segments of the lower lobes
- ☐   C   anterior segments of the upper lobes
- ☐   D   posterior segments of the upper lobes
- ☐   E   the right lung more often than the left

6   A Parkinsonian syndrome may be produced by

- ☐   A   magnesium poisoning
- ☐   B   N-methyl-4-phenyl-1,2,3,6-tetrahydropyridine
- ☐   C   carbon dioxide poisoning
- ☐   D   Wilson's disease
- ☐   E   Huntington's disease

7   Recognized side effects of benzodiazepines include

- ☐   A   confusion
- ☐   B   impaired driving skills
- ☐   C   potentiation of the effects of alcohol
- ☐   D   ataxia
- ☐   E   aplastic anaemia

8   Atrial natriuretic peptide

- ☐   A   is secreted by the left atrium
- ☐   B   receptors are found in the kidney
- ☐   C   stimulates renal sodium reabsorption
- ☐   D   consists of 28 amino acids
- ☐   E   secretion is inhibited in congestive cardiac failure

9   Glibenclamide

- [ ] A   has no biologically active metabolites
- [ ] B   has a shorter half life than chlorpropamide
- [ ] C   stimulates gluconeogenesis
- [ ] D   does not cross the placenta
- [ ] E   is safe in renal impairment

10   Cholestatic jaundice occurs with

- [ ] A   pregnancy
- [ ] B   erythromycin stearate
- [ ] C   verapamil
- [ ] D   prochlorperazine
- [ ] E   amitriptyline

11   The anterior interosseous nerve

- [ ] A   is a branch of the ulnar nerve
- [ ] B   supplies flexor pollicis longus
- [ ] C   supplies abductor pollicis brevis
- [ ] D   supplies extensor pollicis longus
- [ ] E   supplies the first and second lumbricals

12   Evidence for atrio-ventricular dissociation during ventricular tachycardia includes

- [ ] A   occasional cannon 'a' waves in the JVP
- [ ] B   cannon 'a' waves in the JVP at the same rate as ventricular systole
- [ ] C   variable intensity of the first heart sound
- [ ] D   fusion beats on the ECG
- [ ] E   termination by adenosine

13 The following are true of Hantavirus infection:

☐ A it is transmitted by arthropod vectors
☐ B it causes haemorrhagic fever with renal syndrome
☐ C it has been associated with acute respiratory illness
☐ D treatment with ribavarin is of benefit
☐ E it causes nephropathia epidemica

14 The following are typical of syringomyelia:

☐ A Horner's syndrome
☐ B pseudobulbar palsy
☐ C loss of pain and temperature sensation
☐ D loss of proprioception
☐ E loss of reflexes in upper limbs

15 Angiotensin converting enzyme

☐ A is a glycoprotein
☐ B activates bradykinin
☐ C blood concentration may be raised in primary biliary cirrhosis
☐ D is raised in tuberculosis in less than 10% of cases
☐ E levels in active sarcoidosis are unaffected by ACE inhibitor therapy

16 A low serum folate is a common finding in

☐ A tropical sprue
☐ B pernicious anaemia
☐ C megaloblastic anaemia of pregnancy
☐ D myxoedema
☐ E cirrhosis of the liver

17 Recognized features of Wilson's disease include

- ☐ A retinitis pigmentosa
- ☐ B low urinary copper
- ☐ C liver disease resembling chronic active hepatitis
- ☐ D reduced plasma caeruloplasmin
- ☐ E osteomalacia

18 Metformin

- ☐ A is indicated in obese maturity-onset diabetics
- ☐ B stimulates insulin release from the pancreas
- ☐ C does not cause hypoglycaemia
- ☐ D accumulates in renal insufficiency
- ☐ E may cause vitamin B12 deficiency

19 The following are characteristic of renal vasculitis:

- ☐ A macroscopic renal infarction
- ☐ B inactive urinary sediment
- ☐ C eosinophilia
- ☐ D prodrome of systemic illness
- ☐ E progression to end-stage renal failure in over 75%

20 Renin

- ☐ A is synthesized by cells of the distal tubule
- ☐ B cleaves the two N-terminal amino acids of angiotensin I
- ☐ C release is stimulated by a decrease in chloride delivery from the loop of Henle
- ☐ D transcription is stimulated by ACE inhibitors
- ☐ E concentration in blood has a high positive predictive value for renal artery stenosis

21 The following are causes of secondary hyperlipidaemia:

☐ A anorexia nervosa
☐ B chronic renal failure
☐ C hypothyroidism
☐ D steroid therapy
☐ E high alcohol intake

22 In severe paracetamol poisoning

☐ A the hepatotoxin is a metabolite rather than paracetamol itself
☐ B plasma paracetamol concentrations give a useful guide to prognosis
☐ C the earliest evidence of liver damage is a rise in plasma transaminase concentration
☐ D acetylcysteine is effective only if given intravenously
☐ E hepatic coma responds to treatment with neomycin and lactulose

23 Cranial diabetes insipidus is a feature of

☐ A craniopharyngioma
☐ B histiocytosis X
☐ C sarcoidosis
☐ D non-secreting pituitary adenoma
☐ E head injury

24 In polycythaemia rubra vera

☐ A generalized pruritus is typically worse after a hot bath
☐ B a low MCV is a recognized complication
☐ C gout is a recognized complication
☐ D the diagnostic value of raised leucocyte alkaline phosphatase is limited
☐ E splenomegaly is found in 75% of cases

25 The following are true of *E. coli* gastroenteritis:

- ☐ A enterotoxigenic strains are a common cause of travellers' diarrhoea
- ☐ B enteropathogenic strains are associated with the haemolytic uraemic syndrome
- ☐ C enteroadherent strains are non pathogenic
- ☐ D enterohaemorrhagic strains commonly belong to the serotype 0-157
- ☐ E enteroinvasive strains cause a dysenteric illness

26 A urine sodium concentration of 10 mmol/l is likely

- ☐ A following relief of bilateral ureteric obstruction
- ☐ B in severe dehydration
- ☐ C in cranial diabetes insipidus
- ☐ D in a patient with chronic pyelonephritis
- ☐ E in acute tubular necrosis due to burns

27 The following are typical features of Pick's disease:

- ☐ A behavioural disturbance
- ☐ B prominent grasp reflexes
- ☐ C extrapyramidal rigidity
- ☐ D abnormal EEG
- ☐ E familial in approximately 80% of cases

28 Typical features of farmers' lung are

- ☐ A history of exposure to mouldy hay
- ☐ B reduced diffusion capacity
- ☐ C cough with profuse expectoration
- ☐ D pronounced eosinophilia
- ☐ E seasonal incidence May to July

29 The risk of pregnancy despite combined contraceptive steroid usage is increased by concurrent treatment with

- ☐ A diazepam
- ☐ B isoniazid
- ☐ C carbamazepine
- ☐ D phenytoin
- ☐ E rifampicin

30 Splenectomy

- ☐ A results in increased incidence of pneumococcal septicaemia
- ☐ B is a valuable diagnostic procedure in non-Hodgkin's lymphoma
- ☐ C produces blood film appearance of acanthocytes and Howell-Jolly bodies
- ☐ D produces blood film changes which are also seen in coeliac disease
- ☐ E leads to almost invariable remission in hereditary spherocytosis

31 Causes of atrial fibrillation include

- ☐ A hyperthyroidism
- ☐ B recent myocardial infarction
- ☐ C chronic hypertension
- ☐ D cardiac surgery
- ☐ E subdural haematoma

32 In aortic regurgitation

- ☐ A the Austin-Flint murmur is associated with a mitral opening snap
- ☐ B an aortic ejection systolic murmur indicates co-existing aortic stenosis
- ☐ C increasing severity of regurgitation prolongs the murmur
- ☐ D increasing severity of regurgitation lowers diastolic blood pressure
- ☐ E antibiotic prophylaxis is not required

33 Crohn's disease

☐ A presents with fistulae into other organs
☐ B is effectively treated with elemental diet alone
☐ C commonly involves the stomach
☐ D involving the small bowel can be treated with 5-amino salicylic acid
☐ E is more closely associated with sclerosing cholangitis than ulcerative colitis

34 The following are recognised presenting symptoms of carcinoma of the bronchus without metastases:

☐ A tetany
☐ B painful wrists and ankles
☐ C ataxia
☐ D thirst
☐ E increased skin pigmentation

35 Myoclonus is a typical clinical feature of

☐ A Pick's disease
☐ B subacute sclerosing panencephalitis
☐ C primary generalized epilepsy
☐ D post anoxic brain damage
☐ E Creutzfeldt-Jakob disease

36 Carbon dioxide carriage in the blood is

☐ A principally in simple solution
☐ B more than 60% as bicarbonate
☐ C as carbamino compounds in red cells alone
☐ D dependent on the oxygen saturation of haemoglobin
☐ E unaffected in early fibrosing alveolitis

37 *Legionella pneumophila*

☐ A is a Gram-positive bacillus
☐ B infection is associated with lymphopenia
☐ C infection may be diagnosed by urine antigen detection
☐ D causes disease by ingestion of infected water
☐ E causes Pontiac fever

38 The following can cause a ptosis:

☐ A medial medullary lesion
☐ B pontine lesion
☐ C lower motor neurone seventh cranial nerve palsy
☐ D myotonia congenita
☐ E syringobulbia

39 The following may occur after renal transplantation:

☐ A necrosis of the femoral head
☐ B hirsutism
☐ C visual impairment due to macular degeneration
☐ D retardation of growth
☐ E squamous cell carcinoma of the skin

40 Endothelin-1

☐ A is secreted as a prohormone
☐ B selectively constricts the glomerular efferent arteriole
☐ C serum concentration is elevated in heart failure
☐ D is a short acting local vasoconstrictor
☐ E has bronchoconstrictor activity

41 In a study of 54 patients with symptoms of non-ulcer dyspepsia, 27 were treated with bismuth alone and 27 were treated with metronidazole plus amoxycillin. The presence or absence of *H. pylori* infection and a global symptom score (range 0–24) was obtained for each patient both before and after the treatment period.

☐ A if the pre-treatment symptom scores have Normal distribution, the two groups are best compared by use of a nonparametric test

☐ B the post-treatment symptom scores for the two treatment groups can be compared by use of either Student's unpaired t-test or the Mann-Whitney U-test as these two techniques are equivalent

☐ C Student's paired t-test can be used to enhance the change in symptom score within either treatment group only if the median scores are known

☐ D the proportions of patients in the two groups with *H. pylori* infection can be compared by use of a chi-squared test

☐ E a chi-squared test is valid only if all of the expected frequencies are greater than 5

42 The following are true of 'hysteria':

☐ A the physical symptom is produced deliberately
☐ B it may be associated with a depressive illness
☐ C it is associated with 'la belle indifference'
☐ D it characteristically occurs for the first time in middle age
☐ E the physical symptoms and signs closely resemble those of organic disease

43 The following are true:

☐ A restriction fragment length polymorphisms allow a defective gene to be detected only if the gene is known

☐ B oligonucleotide probes can be used to detect a condition caused by a deleted gene

☐ C Down's syndrome may be caused by a translocation

☐ D Gaucher's disease may be diagnosed prenatally

☐ E inherited factor eight deficiency may be diagnosed using a chorionic villus sample

44 Cryptococcal meningitis is characterized by

- ☐ A an abrupt onset
- ☐ B a lymphocytic CSF
- ☐ C negative CSF cryptococcal antigen in 30% of cases
- ☐ D non-communicating hydrocephalus on CT scanning
- ☐ E a tendency to relapses after therapy

45 The sciatic nerve

- ☐ A divides into the tibial and common peroneal nerves at a <u>variable</u> level in the lower limbs
- ☐ B is derived from the L4,5 and S1,2 and 3 spinal nerves
- ☐ C supplies adductor brevis, longus and magnus
- ☐ D supplies quadriceps femoris
- ☐ E supplies gluteus maximus

46 Vesicles are found typically in

- ☐ A pompholyx eczema
- ☐ B exfoliative dermatitis
- ☐ C dermatitis herpetiformis
- ☐ D acute intermittent porphyria
- ☐ E sarcoidosis

47 In patients with sarcoidosis

- ☐ A if there is associated erythema nodosum, the Kveim test is characteristically positive
- ☐ B unilateral hilar adenopathy is a frequent presentation
- ☐ C diffuse pulmonary involvement without any symptoms is a recognized feature
- ☐ D heart failure is usually due to primary myocardial involvement
- ☐ E hypercalcaemia is due to bone involvement

48 In dystrophia myotonica (myotonic dystrophy)

- ☐ A the abnormal gene lies on chromosome 17
- ☐ B the clinical manifestations are usually more severe if the affected parent is male
- ☐ C weakness is initially marked in distal limb musculature
- ☐ D myotonia is most pronounced in the cold
- ☐ E cardiomyopathy is a recognized complication

49 Paroxysmal nocturnal haemoglobinuria

- ☐ A is a hereditary form of haemolytic anaemia
- ☐ B is exacerbated by acidosis
- ☐ C is associated with aplastic anaemia
- ☐ D results from heterologous complement attack
- ☐ E is due to a defect in the glycosyl-phosphatidylinositol anchor

50 Causes of gynaecomastia include

- ☐ A prostatic carcinoma
- ☐ B normal puberty
- ☐ C hypothyroidism
- ☐ D diabetes mellitus
- ☐ E cimetidine

51 Chronic pancreatitis

- ☐ A is associated with hypercalcaemia
- ☐ B may cause portal hypertension
- ☐ C is best diagnosed early by CT scan
- ☐ D produces steatorrhoea when exocrine function falls to 30% or less
- ☐ E is associated with peripheral vascular disease

52　Protein C

- ☐　A　plasma level falls in patients receiving warfarin
- ☐　B　deficiency produces a prolongation in the activated partial thromboplastin time (APTT)
- ☐　C　requires Protein S as a co-factor
- ☐　D　plasma level falls in disseminated intravascular coagulation (DIC)
- ☐　E　potentiates the activity of antithrombin III

53　Fungal arthritis is suggested by

- ☐　A　indolent synovitis
- ☐　B　compromised host
- ☐　C　recent travel in endemic area
- ☐　D　discolouration of synovium
- ☐　E　unpleasant smelling synovial fluid

54　Proliferative diabetic retinopathy

- ☐　A　is treated with laser to the new vessels
- ☐　B　is common at presentation of IDDM
- ☐　C　improves in pregnancy
- ☐　D　is associated with rubeosis iridis
- ☐　E　precludes driving a car

55　A unilateral pontine lesion may produce

- ☐　A　ipsilateral hemiplegia
- ☐　B　diplopia
- ☐　C　pseudobulbar palsy
- ☐　D　ipsilateral third cranial nerve palsy
- ☐　E　ipsilateral upper motor neurone lesion of seventh cranial nerve

56 In chronic constrictive pericarditis

☐ A the patient is breathless at rest
☐ B the jugular venous pulse rises on inspiration
☐ C the jugular venous pulse falls markedly in early diastole
☐ D rapid early ventricular filling may be audible
☐ E the patient is rarely in persistent atrial fibrillation

57 The following drugs may cause haemolytic anaemia

☐ A dapsone
☐ B nifedipine
☐ C methyl dopa
☐ D mefenamic acid
☐ E sulphasalazine

58 Periorbital oedema is a feature of

☐ A Chagas disease
☐ B trichinosis
☐ C gnathostomiasis
☐ D loa-loa infection
☐ E group A streptococcal infection

59 In a normal individual

☐ A 80% of circulating thyroxine is protein bound
☐ B most serum triiodothyronine is produced in the thyroid
☐ C thyroglobulin binds thyroxine in serum
☐ D thyroxine half life is >24 hours
☐ E thyrotrophin (TSH) inhibits thyroid growth

60 *Clostridium difficile*

☐ A   is present in the normal colonic flora of 15–20% of adults
☐ B   colitis is more likely the longer the preceding antibiotic treatment
☐ C   occasionally produces fulminant colitis requiring urgent colectomy
☐ D   produces diagnostic histological changes
☐ E   colitis is best treated with i.v. metronidazole

END OF EXAM 3

Go over your answers until your time is up. Answers and teaching notes are on page 101.

60 questions: Time allowed 2½ hours.
Mark your answers with a tick (True) or a cross (False) in the box provided.
Leave the box blank for 'Don't know'.

1 Calcified extra cardiac lesions on chest X-ray have a recognized association with

- ☐ A asbestosis
- ☐ B farmers' lung
- ☐ C mitral stenosis
- ☐ D silicosis
- ☐ E chickenpox

2 Chorea is a recognized manifestation of

- ☐ A pregnancy
- ☐ B L-dopa medication
- ☐ C choreoacanthosis
- ☐ D hypoparathyroidism
- ☐ E polycythaemia rubra vera

3 Tricyclic antidepressants

- ☐ A are contraindicated in patients with glaucoma
- ☐ B may cause dry mouth
- ☐ C produce prolonged PR and QT intervals on the ECG
- ☐ D are safe in patients anticoagulated with warfarin
- ☐ E are contraindicated in patients with ischaemic heart disease

4 Features of primary hypoparathyroidism include

- ☐ A basal ganglia calcification
- ☐ B carpopedal spasm
- ☐ C serum phosphate 0.5 mmol/l
- ☐ D elevated serum alkaline phosphatase
- ☐ E delayed relaxation of tendon reflexes

5   **Serum K$^+$ 2.5 mmol/l and HCO^{3-} 14 mmol/l suggests**

- ☐   A   acetazolamide treatment
- ☐   B   bulimia
- ☐   C   Conn's syndrome
- ☐   D   uretero-colonic fistula
- ☐   E   methanol poisoning

6   **Hepatitis C**

- ☐   A   is a DNA virus of the herpes type
- ☐   B   is less likely to result in liver cirrhosis than hepatitis B
- ☐   C   is associated with hepatocellular carcinoma
- ☐   D   infection may be complicated by superadded hepatitis D
- ☐   E   is less likely to produce jaundice than hepatitis B

7   **In distinguishing between a C7 nerve root lesion and a radial nerve palsy**

- ☐   A   weakness of triceps is more suggestive of a C7 nerve root lesion
- ☐   B   weakness of brachioradialis indicates a radial nerve palsy
- ☐   C   weakness of wrist flexion suggests a C7 nerve root lesion
- ☐   D   sensory loss affecting the medial aspect of forearm and medial two fingers suggests a C7 nerve root lesion
- ☐   E   an absent brachioradialis reflex does not help to distinguish between a C7 nerve root lesion and a radial nerve palsy

8   **Left atrial myxoma is associated with**

- ☐   A   signs suggesting mitral stenosis
- ☐   B   syncope
- ☐   C   acute pulmonary oedema
- ☐   D   cerebrovascular accident
- ☐   E   increased erythrocyte sedimentation rate

9   *Plasmodium vivax*

- ☐   A   causes quartan malaria
- ☐   B   is associated with relapsing disease
- ☐   C   is often resistant to chloroquine
- ☐   D   is transmitted by Culicine mosquitoes
- ☐   E   infection should be eradicated with primaquine

10   The following diseases are associated with subcortical dementia

- ☐   A   Binswanger's disease
- ☐   B   Alzheimer's disease
- ☐   C   Huntington's disease (chorea)
- ☐   D   Pick's disease
- ☐   E   progressive supranuclear palsy (Steele-Richardson-Olszewski syndrome)

11   Cheyne-Stokes breathing is a recognized feature of

- ☐   A   uraemia
- ☐   B   head injury
- ☐   C   meningitis
- ☐   D   diabetic ketoacidosis
- ☐   E   left ventricular failure

12   Urobilinogen in urine is

- ☐   A   not detectable in health
- ☐   B   distinguished from porphobilinogen by Ehrlich's aldehyde reagent
- ☐   C   diagnostic of intrahepatic obstruction
- ☐   D   increased in pernicious anaemia
- ☐   E   reduced by haemolysis

13 The carcinoid syndrome

- ☐ A frequently responds to octreotide
- ☐ B usually causes mitral valve dysfunction
- ☐ C is invariably fatal within 5 years
- ☐ D causes pallor and sweating
- ☐ E is diagnosed with fasting blood specimens

14 Minoxidil

- ☐ A causes arteriolar vasodilation
- ☐ B accumulates dangerously in renal failure
- ☐ C must not be used with a loop diuretic
- ☐ D increases growth of body hair
- ☐ E causes flattening or inversion of the T-wave on the ECG

15 In a patient with renal impairment, the following would indicate acute, as opposed to chronic renal failure

- ☐ A recent commencement of captopril for hypertensive treatment
- ☐ B Hb of 6 g/dl with RBC fragmentation and reticulocytosis
- ☐ C renal bipolar diameters of 13 cm
- ☐ D presence of an abdominal aortic aneurysm
- ☐ E recurrent urinary infections

16 Correct descriptions of chemotherapeutic agents include

- ☐ A cyclophosphamide: alkylating agent
- ☐ B methotrexate: folic acid antagonist
- ☐ C azathioprine: vinca alkaloid
- ☐ D vinblastine: pyrimidine analogue
- ☐ E cytosine arabinoside: purine analogue

17 Transforming growth factor beta

- ☐ A promotes wound healing
- ☐ B is released from platelets during degranulation
- ☐ C has one active isoform
- ☐ D has autocrine activity
- ☐ E stimulates lymphocyte proliferation

18 In hypertrophic obstructive cardiomyopathy (HOCM)

- ☐ A atrial fibrillation indicates a poor prognosis
- ☐ B the characteristic murmur is loudest in the aortic area
- ☐ C propranolol therapy prevents sudden death
- ☐ D trinitrin reduces outflow obstruction
- ☐ E there are characteristic echocardiographic findings

19 Recognized features of digoxin toxicity include

- ☐ A weight loss
- ☐ B unilateral gynaecomastia
- ☐ C diplopia
- ☐ D ventricular fibrillation
- ☐ E delirium

20 Features of Cushing's disease include

- ☐ A hypertension
- ☐ B psychiatric symptoms
- ☐ C tall stature in children
- ☐ D hypertrichosis
- ☐ E macrocytic anaemia

21 The following haematological disorders are seen in association with infection by HIV:

- ☐ A atypical lymphocytes in the peripheral blood
- ☐ B immune thrombocytopenic purpura (ITP)
- ☐ C megaloblastic erythroblasts in the bone marrow in the absence of vitamin B12/folate deficiency
- ☐ D positive lupus anticoagulant screen
- ☐ E monocytopenia

22 The following are features of encephalitis:

- ☐ A herpes simplex encephalitis is usually caused by HSV 2
- ☐ B chickenpox encephalitis typically coincides with the onset of rash
- ☐ C herpes simplex predominantly affects the temporal lobes
- ☐ D mycoplasma encephalitis only occurs in the immunocompromised
- ☐ E Japanese B encephalitis is preventable by vaccination

23 Hyperuricaemia occurs in

- ☐ A Lesch-Nyhan syndrome
- ☐ B polycythaemia rubra vera
- ☐ C primary hyperparathyroidism
- ☐ D starvation
- ☐ E thyrotoxicosis

24 A unilateral lesion in the midbrain can produce

- ☐ A ipsilateral sixth cranial nerve palsy
- ☐ B contralateral hemiplegia
- ☐ C contralateral ataxia
- ☐ D ipsilateral Horner's syndrome
- ☐ E pseudobulbar palsy

25 Bilateral basal crackles are a typical finding in the following

- [ ] A emphysema due to alpha-1 anti-trypsin deficiency
- [ ] B bronchiectasis following childhood whooping cough
- [ ] C pulmonary sarcoidosis
- [ ] D fibrosing alveolitis
- [ ] E acute attack of asthma

26 Diazepam

- [ ] A is associated with development of tolerance to its actions
- [ ] B causes physical dependence (addiction)
- [ ] C inhibits warfarin metabolism
- [ ] D impairs GABA facilitated inhibitory synaptic transmission
- [ ] E has no active metabolites

27 Marrow trephine biopsy is more satisfactory than marrow aspiration in the diagnosis of

- [ ] A aplastic anaemia
- [ ] B sideroblastic anaemia
- [ ] C macrocytic anaemia
- [ ] D marrow involvement in Hodgkin's disease
- [ ] E myelosclerosis

28 Benign intracranial hypertension (BIH)

- [ ] A usually occurs in thin young females
- [ ] B may be caused by hypervitaminosis D
- [ ] C causes enlargement of the blind spot
- [ ] D may cause a sixth cranial nerve palsy
- [ ] E is characterized by normal or enlarged lateral ventricles on CT or MR scan

29 Oxygen debt

- [ ] A may be six times the basal oxygen consumption
- [ ] B in trained athletes is greater than in an untrained person for a given amount of exertion
- [ ] C is limited by an increase in pH
- [ ] D is incurred because blood cannot be delivered to the muscle at a high enough rate
- [ ] E is possible because muscle is capable of anaerobic metabolism

30 Endothelium derived relaxation factor

- [ ] A acts via specific receptors on vascular smooth muscle cells
- [ ] B is nitric oxide
- [ ] C is formed from L-citrulline
- [ ] D is stored in the endoplasmic reticulum of endothelial cells
- [ ] E increases intracellular cyclic GMP

31 Significant elevation of plasma gastrin level is found

- [ ] A after massive small bowel resection
- [ ] B in patients treated with omeprazole
- [ ] C in chronic renal failure
- [ ] D in duodenal ulcer
- [ ] E in multiple endocrine neoplasia type IIB

32 In leptospirosis

- [ ] A conjunctivitis is a frequent early symptom
- [ ] B the onset is characteristically abrupt
- [ ] C splenomegaly is found in the majority of patients
- [ ] D the transaminases are markedly elevated
- [ ] E the diagnosis is best made by serology

33 Characteristic features of early diffuse interstitial fibrosis include

☐ A cyanosis at rest
☐ B reduced vital capacity
☐ C reduced FEV1/FVC ratio
☐ D bilateral reticular shadowing on chest X-ray
☐ E reduced pulmonary diffusing capacity

34 The following are true of transient global amnesia (TGA):

☐ A it usually occurs in individuals over the age of 40
☐ B personal identity is typically preserved
☐ C there is no associated reduction of consciousness
☐ D it has a low recurrence rate
☐ E it is typically associated with precipitating factors

35 G Proteins

☐ A phosphorylate guanosine diphosphate
☐ B include Ras oncoproteins
☐ C deactivation occurs via hydrolysis
☐ D are transmembrane signal-receptor molecules
☐ E are found in all cell types

36 In a clinical trial of a new drug, the following results were obtained

	Drug	Placebo
Improved	46 patients	34 patients
Not improved	14 patients	26 patients

☐ A the superiority of the drug over the placebo is so obvious that formal statistical testing is unnecessary
☐ B if a test of significance were required, computation of the Pearson coefficient of linear correlation would be appropriate
☐ C the data could be evaluated by computing a chi-squared statistic
☐ D the data could be evaluated by computing Student's t-test
☐ E the data could now be submitted to sequential analysis

37 The following are true of suicide:

- ☐ A two-thirds of those who die by suicide have told someone of their intention
- ☐ B asking about suicidal intent will increase the risk of suicide
- ☐ C patients with chronical physical illness are at increased risk
- ☐ D it is associated with alcohol abuse
- ☐ E it is most common in young women

38 In the cell cycle

- ☐ A cytoplasmic cleavage occurs in G2
- ☐ B DNA is replicated in S phase
- ☐ C organelles are synthesised in metaphase
- ☐ D interphase occupies the largest part of the cell cycle
- ☐ E the chromatids separate in anaphase

39 In syphilis

- ☐ A the majority of patients with secondary syphilis have mucosal ulcers
- ☐ B accelerated progression may occur in HIV-positive patients
- ☐ C the TPHA test usually becomes negative after treatment
- ☐ D phenoxy methyl penicillin is the treatment of choice
- ☐ E condylomata accuminata occur in the perianal region

40 The femoral nerve supplies

- ☐ A gluteus minimus
- ☐ B vastus lateralis
- ☐ C skin of the lateral aspect of the thigh
- ☐ D gastrocnemius
- ☐ E hamstring muscles (semitendinosus, semimembranosus and biceps)

41 Urticaria may be associated with

- ☐ A *Strongyloides* infection
- ☐ B opiate drugs
- ☐ C paracetamol
- ☐ D systemic lupus erythematosus
- ☐ E pityriasis rosea

42 *Pneumocystis carinii* infection

- ☐ A is the most common opportunist lung infection in AIDS
- ☐ B responds to treatment with co-trimoxazole (Septrin)
- ☐ C can usually be diagnosed by bronchoalveolar lavage
- ☐ D should be treated with prednisolone if moderate or severe
- ☐ E now has a first exposure mortality of less than 15%

43 The following are typical clinical manifestations of myasthenia gravis:

- ☐ A diplopia
- ☐ B dysphasia
- ☐ C absent tendon reflexes
- ☐ D distal limb weakness
- ☐ E fatiguability

44 Bicuspid aortic valves

- ☐ A rarely calcify
- ☐ B are associated with Turner's syndrome
- ☐ C are associated with coarctation of the aorta
- ☐ D occur in 0.01% of the population
- ☐ E are the most common cause of aortic stenosis in the over 80s

45 Alport's syndrome

- ☐ A is autosomal recessive
- ☐ B is due to a mutation of the Goodpasture antigen
- ☐ C results in basement membrane changes in the eye
- ☐ D can recur in renal transplants
- ☐ E is associated with tracheobronchial leiomyomatosis

46 At the female menopause

- ☐ A the patient has her greatest bone mass
- ☐ B oestrogen secretion causes hot flushes
- ☐ C myocardial infarction is common
- ☐ D bowel transit time increases
- ☐ E serum FSH is higher than serum LH

47 The irritable bowel syndrome is associated with

- ☐ A dysuria
- ☐ B a characteristic pattern of abnormal colonic motility
- ☐ C recent salmonella gastroenteritis
- ☐ D non-ulcer dyspepsia
- ☐ E headache

48 Haemophilia A

- ☐ A may be unassociated with a family history
- ☐ B commonly presents with spontaneous purpura
- ☐ C results in prolongation of the activated partial thromboplastin time (APTT) and prothrombin time (PT)
- ☐ D characteristically becomes less severe with advancing age
- ☐ E is associated with a normal bleeding time

49   Indications for hypouricaemic therapy include

☐   A   tophi
☐   B   bone erosion
☐   C   urate levels at upper limit of normal
☐   D   a single, severe attack
☐   E   nephrosclerosis

50   Microalbuminuria in a diabetic patient

☐   A   is best assessed with a 24 hour urine sample
☐   B   is reduced by ACE inhibition
☐   C   follows the development of hypertension
☐   D   indicates the presence of proliferative retinopathy
☐   E   predicts ischaemic heart disease in NIDDM

51   In Parkinson's disease

☐   A   the onset of symptoms is typically before the age of 40
☐   B   tremor is most pronounced on sustained posture
☐   C   rigidity in the upper limbs is most pronounced in the flexor
          muscles
☐   D   gait is typically broad based
☐   E   urinary incontinence is an early clinical feature

52   In left ventricular failure

☐   A   alveolar PCO_2 is increased
☐   B   carbon monoxide diffusion capacity is reduced
☐   C   pulmonary venous pressure is raised
☐   D   left ventricular end-diastolic pressure is reduced
☐   E   basal crepitations are heard before chest X-ray changes are seen

53 The following drugs are excreted mainly in the form of glucuronide or sulphate conjugates

- ☐ A warfarin
- ☐ B temazepam
- ☐ C isoniazid
- ☐ D paracetamol
- ☐ E phenytoin

54 The following antiviral therapies are of proven benefit

- ☐ A amantadine for treatment of influenza A
- ☐ B intravenous acyclovir in chickenpox pneumonitis
- ☐ C zidovudine (AZT) in asymptomatic HIV infection with CD4 count >500 x 10⁶/l
- ☐ D interferon in chronic hepatitis C
- ☐ E ribavarin in lassa fever

55 Unilateral exophthalmos is a feature of

- ☐ A Wegener's granulomatosis
- ☐ B orbital tumour
- ☐ C cigarette smoking
- ☐ D contralateral Horner's syndrome
- ☐ E Graves' disease

56 Malabsorption of fat due to bile acid deficiency occurs in

- ☐ A Crohn's disease
- ☐ B radiation enteritis
- ☐ C cystic fibrosis
- ☐ D coeliac disease
- ☐ E giardiasis

57 Cryoglobulins

- ☐ A are usually IgG or IgM, seldom IgA
- ☐ B are seen in myeloma
- ☐ C are rarely polyclonal
- ☐ D are associated with urticaria
- ☐ E precipitate reversibly at low temperature

58 Haemopoietic growth factors

- ☐ A act on colony forming units
- ☐ B include interleukin 3
- ☐ C are members of the immunoglobulin superfamily
- ☐ D are encoded for by genes on chromosome 3
- ☐ E do not affect mature cell function

59 The following are features of unilateral renal artery stenosis

- ☐ A hypokalaemic alkalosis
- ☐ B renal glycosuria
- ☐ C normochromic, normocytic anaemia
- ☐ D treatment with captopril results in a rise in blood urea
- ☐ E increased concentration of radiographic contrast on the contralateral side

60 The following are Schneiderian first rank symptoms of schizophrenia:

- ☐ A thought insertion
- ☐ B visual hallucinations
- ☐ C suicidal ideas
- ☐ D passivity phenomena
- ☐ E thought broadcast

END OF EXAM 4

Go over your answers until your time is up. Answers and teaching notes are on page 113.

PRACTICE EXAM 5

60 questions: Time allowed 2½ hours.
Mark your answers with a tick (True) or a cross (False) in the box provided.
Leave the box blank for 'Don't know'.

1   A lesion of the common peroneal nerve may

- ☐ A   be produced by a fracture of the neck of fibula
- ☐ B   cause weakness of foot plantar flexion
- ☐ C   abolish foot inversion
- ☐ D   cause loss of sensation affecting skin over the medial aspect of lower leg
- ☐ E   cause loss of ankle reflex

2   In the skin

- ☐ A   the bullous pemphigoid antigen is thought to be a component of the desmosome
- ☐ B   Langerhans cells are important antigen presenting cells within the dermis
- ☐ C   eccrine sweat glands are innervated by adrenergic sympathetic nerve fibres
- ☐ D   melanin is found within melanocytes and keratinocytes
- ☐ E   sebaceous glands are androgen sensitive

3   Pulmonary eosinophilia is a recognized feature of

- ☐ A   nitrofurantoin ingestion
- ☐ B   Loffler's syndrome
- ☐ C   filarial infection
- ☐ D   Wegener's granulomatosis
- ☐ E   Churg-Strauss syndrome

4   The following are true of Duchenne muscular dystrophy:

- ☐ A   it is inherited as an X-linked recessive disorder
- ☐ B   limb weakness usually affects distal musculature
- ☐ C   limb contractures are an early clinical manifestation
- ☐ D   eyes, face and bulbar musculature are usually spared
- ☐ E   EMGs show a typically neuropathic appearance

5   Recognized features of mitral regurgitation include

- [ ] A   loud first heart sound
- [ ] B   mid-systolic click followed by late systolic murmur
- [ ] C   third heart sound
- [ ] D   pansystolic murmur and apical thrill with ECG evidence of a recent posterior infarct
- [ ] E   reversed splitting of the second sound

6   In multiple sclerosis

- [ ] A   there is reduced MHC class II expression in the CNS
- [ ] B   helper T cells are found in acute lesions
- [ ] C   saltatory conduction is normal
- [ ] D   oligodendrocytes proliferate
- [ ] E   the blood brain barrier is impaired

7   In Turner's syndrome

- [ ] A   45 XO karyotype is universal
- [ ] B   tall stature prepubertally is characteristic
- [ ] C   there is poor breast development
- [ ] D   serum FSH is high in the adult
- [ ] E   uterine agenesis is characteristic

8   Ascites is a feature of

- [ ] A   syndrome of inappropriate antidiuretic hormone secretion
- [ ] B   mesothelioma
- [ ] C   acute pericarditis
- [ ] D   marasmus
- [ ] E   hepatocellular carcinoma

9   The following are recognized complications of heparin therapy:

- [ ] A   thrombosis
- [ ] B   osteomalacia
- [ ] C   hirsutism
- [ ] D   thrombocytopenia
- [ ] E   teratogenesis

10   Diseases associated with hypermobility include

- [ ] A   Marfan's syndrome
- [ ] B   acromegaly
- [ ] C   Paget's disease
- [ ] D   amyloidosis
- [ ] E   Wilson's disease

11   Diabetic maculopathy

- [ ] A   is more common in NIDDM than IDDM
- [ ] B   impairs peripheral vision
- [ ] C   is treated by panretinal photocoagulation
- [ ] D   is characterized by drusen at the macula
- [ ] E   causes painful visual loss

12   The following favour a lesion of the cerebral cortex rather than of the brain stem:

- [ ] A   dysarthria
- [ ] B   diplopia
- [ ] C   dysphasia
- [ ] D   hemianopia
- [ ] E   extensor plantar response

13 Pericarditis is a recognized complication of

- ☐ A chronic renal failure
- ☐ B hypothyroidism
- ☐ C reflux oesophagitis
- ☐ D acute rheumatic fever
- ☐ E subarachnoid haemorrhage

14 Antagonists at beta-adrenoceptors commonly produce

- ☐ A cold extremities
- ☐ B delayed recovery from hypoglycaemia
- ☐ C enhancement of physiological tremor
- ☐ D nightmares
- ☐ E increased gastrointestinal haemorrhage in patients with portal hypertension

15 In a patient with a fever a neutrophil leucocytosis (>10 x 10⁹/l) makes the following more likely:

- ☐ A brucellosis
- ☐ B amoebic liver abscess
- ☐ C malaria
- ☐ D dengue fever
- ☐ E typhoid fever

16 The following are recognized features of hypothyroidism:

- ☐ A menorrhagia
- ☐ B ascites
- ☐ C cerebellar ataxia
- ☐ D clubbing
- ☐ E normochromic anaemia

17 *Helicobacter pylori*

- ☐ A is a Gram-positive *Campylobacter*-like organism
- ☐ B produces the enzyme urease
- ☐ C induces erosive antral gastritis
- ☐ D can be found in 75% of patients with a duodenal ulcer
- ☐ E can be diagnosed by a hydrogen breath test

18 Hypocomplementaemia is a feature of

- ☐ A acute pancreatitis
- ☐ B membranous nephropathy
- ☐ C systemic lupus erythematosus
- ☐ D pregnancy
- ☐ E cryoglobulinaemia

19 Apoptosis

- ☐ A causes necrotic cell death
- ☐ B is involved in embryological remodelling
- ☐ C releases proinflammatory mediators
- ☐ D is characterized by condensation of nuclear chromatin T
- ☐ E is associated with endonuclease activation

20 The ureter

- ☐ A contains circular and longitudinal smooth muscle arranged in spirals
- ☐ B is lined with columnar epithelium
- ☐ C receives its sympathetic nerve supply from L2, L3 and L4
- ☐ D develops from the mesonephric duct
- ☐ E radiologically lies on the tips of the transverse processes of the lumbar vertebrae

21 Puerperal psychosis

- [ ] A is more frequent in primiparous women
- [ ] B usually begins in the first two days after delivery
- [ ] C recurrence in subsequent pregnancies is the rule
- [ ] D usually has an insidious onset
- [ ] E normally has a good prognosis

22 The following typically appear in the anterior mediastinum

- [ ] A syphilitic aortic aneurysm
- [ ] B dermoid tumour
- [ ] C thymoma
- [ ] D neuroblastoma
- [ ] E neurofibroma

23 In a 70-year-old man with tremor of the upper limbs, essential tremor rather than Parkinson's disease is more likely to be the cause if

- [ ] A the tremor is worst at rest
- [ ] B the tremor is relieved with alcohol
- [ ] C the tremor is exacerbated by anxiety
- [ ] D the tremor is predominantly postural
- [ ] E there is rigidity

24 Benzodiazepine anxiolytics

- [ ] A are mainly metabolised to sulphate conjugates
- [ ] B have no active metabolites
- [ ] C differ significantly in their duration of action
- [ ] D differ significantly in their sedative effects relative to anxiolytic activity
- [ ] E increase body sway

25   Intact parathyroid hormone

- ☐ A   levels are increased in the hypercalcaemia of sarcoidosis
- ☐ B   concentration is low in primary hyperparathyroidism
- ☐ C   can be measured by immunoradiometric assay
- ☐ D   inhibits renal 1-alpha hydroxylase
- ☐ E   consists of 52 amino acids

26   A serum bicarbonate concentration of 34 mmol/l is consistent with

- ☐ A   cor pulmonale
- ☐ B   21-hydroxylase deficiency
- ☐ C   the observation of carpopedal spasm
- ☐ D   ureterosigmoidostomy
- ☐ E   primary hyperparathyroidism

27   Hepatic encephalopathy may be precipitated by

- ☐ A   metabolic alkalosis
- ☐ B   therapeutic paracentesis
- ☐ C   concurrent treatment with omeprazole
- ☐ D   intravenous 0.9% saline
- ☐ E   intravenous salt poor albumin

28   The following are true of pseudobulbar palsy:

- ☐ A   the gag reflex is usually absent
- ☐ B   the tongue is wasted
- ☐ C   the jaw jerk is usually brisk
- ☐ D   it may be caused by a syrinx extending from the cord into the medulla oblongata
- ☐ E   it is usually due to cerebrovascular disease

29 Infective endocarditis

☐ A is a recognized cause of glomerulonephritis
☐ B when due to *Streptococcus faecalis* should be treated with intravenous benzyl penicillin alone
☐ C is commonly seen in patients with an atrial septal defect and no other cardiac lesion
☐ D is confirmed or excluded by a normal echocardiograph
☐ E may follow sigmoidoscopy

30 The following are true of hepatitis C virus:

☐ A chronic carriage is associated with hepatoma
☐ B it is sexually transmissible
☐ C it is an RNA virus
☐ D infection is confirmed by a positive hepatitis C antigen test
☐ E chronic carriers may benefit from treatment with interferon

31 The following are true of Alzheimer's disease:

☐ A behavioural disturbance is an early clinical manifestation
☐ B extensor plantar responses and myoclonus are early clinical features
☐ C the EEG is usually normal
☐ D it is associated with a predominantly frontal cortical distribution of pathology
☐ E it is usually familial

32 Lung compliance is

☐ A reduced by pulmonary congestion
☐ B a measure of change in lung volume per unit change in airway pressure
☐ C decreased by emphysema
☐ D approximately half in a person with one lung
☐ E determined by use of a peak flow meter

33   A falling haemoglobin with a 20% reticulocyte count may be due to

☐   A   menorrhagia
☐   B   congenital spherocytosis
☐   C   sideroblastic anaemia
☐   D   lead
☐   E   methyl dopa

34   Features of acute intermittent porphyria include

☐   A   more women than men affected
☐   B   increased urinary porphobilinogen
☐   C   photosensitive rash in 25%
☐   D   radial nerve palsy
☐   E   hypernatraemia

35   Sulphasalazine

☐   A   absorption is virtually complete
☐   B   is effective by enema in inflammatory bowel disease
☐   C   inhibits prostaglandin synthesis
☐   D   has caused agranulocytosis
☐   E   reduces fertility

36   Dosages of the following drugs should be reduced in patients with a GFR of less than 20 ml/min

☐   A   enalapril
☐   B   methyl prednisolone
☐   C   metronidazole
☐   D   nifedipine
☐   E   digoxin

37 Adhesion molecules

☐ A are not present on eosinophils
☐ B form tight junctions between cells
☐ C include leucocyte integrins
☐ D are upregulated in inflammatory diseases
☐ E prevent monocyte transmigration

38 The right coronary artery

☐ A originates from the right coronary sinus and lies in the right atrio-ventricular groove
☐ B typically supplies the inferior aspect of the left ventricle
☐ C typically gives rise to the artery to the A-V node
☐ D gives rise to the posterior descending coronary artery in the majority of patients
☐ E occlusion has occurred in the majority of patients with right ventricular infarction and failure

39 Enterohepatic recirculation makes an important contribution to the bioavailability of the following drugs:

☐ A ethinyloestradiol ·
☐ B diazepam
☐ C warfarin .
☐ D phenytoin
☐ E lithium

40 Competitive enzyme inhibitors include

☐ A metyrapone
☐ B finasteride
☐ C enalaprilat
☐ D pralidoxime
☐ E pyridostigmine

41 In phaeochromocytoma

- ☐ A 50% of tumours are extra-adrenal
- ☐ B diarrhoea is common
- ☐ C IVP offers the best tumour localization
- ☐ D medullary thyroid cancer may be associated
- ☐ E urgent beta blockade is essential

42 Thalassaemia major

- ☐ A is a cause of neonatal jaundice
- ☐ B is a cause of short stature
- ☐ C results in a shortened life-span
- ☐ D is an autosomal recessive condition
- ☐ E results in a bossed forehead

43 *Candida albicans*

- ☐ A may cause endophthalmitis
- ☐ B infection is encouraged by renal glycosuria
- ☐ C responds to griseofulvin when affecting the nail bed
- ☐ D causing deep infection is more likely with lymphopenia
- ☐ E endocarditis most commonly involves the tricuspid valve

44 Features of lithium poisoning include

- ☐ A constipation
- ☐ B inappropriate ADH secretion
- ☐ C cerebellar signs
- ☐ D hypokalaemia
- ☐ E coma

45 The following associations are correct in pulmonary disease:

☐ A basal fibrosis and ankylosing spondylitis
☐ B pleurisy with effusion and Sjogren's syndrome
☐ C basal pneumonia and systemic sclerosis
☐ D chylothorax and yellow nails
☐ E lymphangitis – carcinomatosa and carcinoma of the pancreas

46 The following are typical of a unilateral lesion affecting the medial aspect of the medulla oblongata:

☐ A ipsilateral twelfth cranial nerve palsy
☐ B contralateral hemiplegia
☐ C ipsilateral loss of touch and joint position sense
☐ D ipsilateral Horner's syndrome
☐ E ipsilateral ataxia

47 ST depression on ECG is a feature of

☐ A digitalis toxicity
☐ B hypertension
☐ C patients with cardiac syndrome X on exertion
☐ D chronic pericarditis
☐ E hypokalaemia

48 Slow acetylators are more prone to the following adverse drug effect:

☐ A hypertensive crisis with hydralazine
☐ B hepatitis with isoniazid
☐ C nausea and vomiting with sulphasalazine
☐ D peripheral neuropathy with isoniazid
☐ E systemic lupus syndrome with hydralazine

49 Characteristic features of acute falciparum malaria include

- [ ] A splenomegaly
- [ ] B rigors every 72 hours
- [ ] C eosinophilia
- [ ] D renal failure
- [ ] E recurrence of symptoms after one year in untreated survivors

50 Recognized features of Paget's disease of bone include

- [ ] A hypercalcaemia
- [ ] B nerve deafness
- [ ] C angioid streaks in the retina
- [ ] D brain stem compression
- [ ] E osteopenia

51 The following conditions are transmissible spongiform encephalopathies (prion diseases):

- [ ] A subacute sclerosing panencephalitis (SSPE)
- [ ] B Creutzfeldt-Jakob disease (CJD)
- [ ] C Gerstmann-Straussler-Sheinker disease (GSSD)
- [ ] D Kuru
- [ ] E progressive multifocal leucoencephalopathy (PML)

52 In extrinsic allergic alveolitis

- [ ] A the most common sign is fine crackles
- [ ] B precipitating antibodies are diagnostic
- [ ] C there may be asymptomatic pulmonary insufficiency for several years
- [ ] D rheumatoid factor is positive in 30%
- [ ] E systemic symptoms typically occur within 20 minutes of exposure to organic dusts

53 Pancytopenia may be caused by

- ☐ A folic acid deficiency
- ☐ B paroxysmal nocturnal haemoglobinuria
- ☐ C brucellosis
- ☐ D acute myeloblastic leukaemia
- ☐ E haemosiderosis

54 Bilateral facial weakness is a feature of

- ☐ A myasthenia gravis
- ☐ B myotonic dystrophy
- ☐ C sarcoidosis
- ☐ D Guillain-Barré syndrome
- ☐ E a unilateral pontine lesion

55 Pleural effusions

- ☐ A are a common feature of *Pneumocystis carinii* pneumonia
- ☐ B may be blood stained following pulmonary embolus
- ☐ C in asbestosis are almost always due to a mesothelioma
- ☐ D characteristically have a low glucose content in rheumatoid arthritis
- ☐ E usually respond to steroid therapy in SLE

56 Erythropoietin

- ☐ A is only produced in the kidney
- ☐ B production increases in response to hypoxia
- ☐ C therapy is associated with hypertension
- ☐ D acts on the colony forming units of the erythroid series in the bone marrow
- ☐ E is produced in an active and inactive isoform

57 **An article in a medical journal states that in a study of gestational age at birth and neurological development at 12 months of age, r was found to be +0.56 and p<0.001.**

☐ A   r is the correlation coefficient of probability
☐ B   there is a negative association between gestational age and neurological development
☐ C   there is a significant relationship between gestational age and neurological development
☐ D   pre-term birth causes an inhibition in neurological development
☐ E   the small value of p means that too few infants were studied

58 **The following are associated with dementia:**

☐ A   pernicious anaemia
☐ B   hypervitaminosis A
☐ C   pellagra
☐ D   porphyria
☐ E   Wilson's disease

59 **In genetic technology**

☐ A   a codon consists of three nucleotides
☐ B   introns are transcribed into messenger RNA
☐ C   endonucleases polymerise DNA fragments
☐ D   thymidine is not found in messenger RNA
☐ E   transcription can be measured by Northern blotting

60 **In tuberculosis**

☐ A   multiple drug resistance only occurs in the immunocompromised
☐ B   vertebral body destruction is an early radiological sign in spinal disease
☐ C   pyrazinamide should be given for six months
☐ D   the response to treatment in HIV-positive patients is poor
☐ E   steroids should be given for pericardial disease

END OF EXAM 5

Go over your answers until your time is up. Answers and teaching notes are on page 126.

ANSWERS AND TEACHING NOTES

ANSWERS TO PRACTICE EXAM 1

1 **C D**
Proto-oncogenes are normal cellular genes that control a variety of processes associated with cell growth and differentiation. They are transiently
stimulated by growth factors. Oncogenes are altered or over-expressed
versions of proto-oncogene counterparts that lack regulatory constraints
and do not need external activation signals. Oncogenes are associated with
the development of a wide variety of human tumours.

2 **A C E**
B is false – it is hoped that the sample mean will be equal to the population
mean, but in reality they are rarely exactly equal. D is false – the median is
equal to the mean when the data are normally distributed.

3 **A B D E**
The central clinical features of anorexia nervosa are low body weight (15%
below normal weight), distorted body image and amenorrhoea. Vomiting
and laxative abuse may lead to hypokalaemia. Several hormonal abnormalities may occur: raised growth hormone, raised plasma cortisol with
loss of diurnal variation, low gonadotrophins and low triiodothyronine.
There are numerous medical complications such as bradycardia, hypotension, cardiac arrhythmias, oedema, osteoporosis, hypothermia, salivary
gland enlargement, pancreatitis, hypoglycaemia and erosion of tooth
enamel. Depressed mood is common.

4 **B C D**
A condition is dominant if the disease is expressed despite normal copies
of the gene being present on one chromosome; i.e. heterozygotes have the
disease as well as homozygotes. A condition is recessive if the genes on
both of the chromosomes have to be abnormal for the disease to be
expressed. Wilson's disease and Erb's muscular dystrophy are recessive,
while arachnodactyly, familial polyposis coli and tuberous sclerosis are
dominantly inherited.

5 **A C D**
Approximately 30% of patients develop an acute febrile illness in association with seroconversion. Common features are a maculopapular rash, oral
ulceration and generalized lymphadenopathy. A rise in indicators of viral
replication occur with the illness and antibody tests usually become
positive 2–6 weeks after the onset. Increased severity of the illness is
associated with a poorer prognosis.

6   B C

Brachialis is supplied by the musculocutaneous nerve (C5,6). The radial nerve (C5,6,7,8) supplies brachioradialis. Abductor pollicis brevis and first lumbrical are supplied by median nerve (C6,7,8, T1). Sensory loss due to a radial nerve lesion affects skin over the lateral aspect of the dorsal hand surface.

7   D

Seborrhoeic warts may occur in any area where there are pilosebaceous follicles, but they are seen predominantly on the face and trunk. They are non-infective and best removed by curettage or cryotherapy. Large numbers of seborrhoeic warts may appear suddenly together with pruritus in association with an internal malignancy (Leser-Trelat sign). Cowden disease or multiple hamartoma syndrome, an autosomal dominant condition is characterized by multiple trichilemmomas, buccal papillomatosis, lipomas and angiomas in association with a predisposition to carcinoma of the breast and thyroid.

8   A B C E

Drug resistance remains low in the UK (2-3% in the non-treated Caucasian population) but is much higher in certain areas of the USA, especially New York. Large tuberculous pleural effusions respond well to a combination of chemotherapy and prednisolone.

9   A E

The presence of antibodies to acetylcholine receptors is specific to myasthenia gravis. Antibodies to striated muscle are associated with the presence of a thymoma. Tendon and pupillary reflexes are normal. Large doses of anticholinesterases may precipitate a cholinergic crisis. This can be distinguished from a myasthenic crisis by the presence of cholinergic features of sweating, salivation, diarrhoea and miosis.

10   B E

Innocent murmurs tend to be ejection systolic. Diastolic or pansystolic murmurs are pathological. An exceptional innocent murmur is a venous hum, which is continuous and often occurs in children. It may disappear on neck vein compression or on lying down. An innocent pulmonary flow murmur is common in children. A thrill or associated added sound makes any murmur unlikely to be innocent.

11   A C D

Hepatitis B is a small DNA virus consisting of genomic DNA, core protein and surface protein. The core gene encodes for both core antigen and a cleavage product e antigen, which is a good marker of active viral replication. Pre S, which is closely associated with the surface antigen viral envelope, has specific attachment sites for hepatocytes. Interferon inhibits virus replication. Hepatitis D is a defective virus that requires hepatitis B virus to supply envelope proteins and can only infect man in the presence of HBV.

12 A B

21 Hydroxylase deficiency leads to a block in conversion from 17 hydroxyprogesterone to 11 deoxycortisol (glucocorticoid pathway) and from progesterone to 11 deoxycorticosterone (mineralocorticoid pathway). Elevated plasma levels of the steroids proximal to the block (progesterone and 17 OH-progesterone) and their urinary metabolites (pregnanetriol) are characteristic. Accumulated 17 OH-progesterone is diverted to androstenedione with subsequent conversion to testosterone, which causes clitoromegaly in the female foetus and early enlargement of the genitalia in boys. In salt-losers, there is impaired mineralocorticoid action and thus reflex increase in renin secretion.

13 A C D

Other well recognized causes of intestinal pseudo-obstruction (i.e. no mechanical lesion but clinical and radiological features of obstruction) include progressive systemic sclerosis, diabetes mellitus, hypothyroidism and chronic phenothiazine therapy. Rarely, it is the presenting manifestation of occult neoplasm, either small cell lung cancer or phaeochromocytoma.

14 A B E

In A there is hormonal suppression of normal cells by leukaemic cells and mechanical 'crowding out' in the bone marrow. In B thrombocytopenia may be an initial manifestation. Septicaemia induces consumption by immune complexes, complement activation and direct toxaemia. Massive transfusion produces thrombocytopenia by dilution.

15 A C E

Pericarditis is a common feature of rheumatic disease. The clinical consequences are usually slight. Acute pericarditis may predate diagnosis of underlying disease, particularly in rheumatoid arthritis and SLE.

16 E

Whereas pruritus and in particular genital pruritus is a common feature of diabetes mellitus, it is not diagnostic. Similarly, diabetes insipidus, hypercalcaemia and hypokalaemia may all present with polyuria. Glycosuria is most commonly due to diabetes but renal glycosuria (low threshold) must be considered. The fasting venous plasma glucose must exceed 7.8 mmol/l to confirm the diagnosis and the value 2 hours after a 75 g oral glucose tolerance test must be >11.0 mmol/l. Note that the diagnostic values differ according to whether glucose is measured in capillary whole blood, venous whole blood or venous plasma — the latter is used most commonly in the UK.

17 None correct

Thrombosis of the posterior inferior cerebellar artery or vertebral artery may cause infarction of the lateral medulla oblongata (Wallenberg's syndrome). It gives rise to ipsilateral Horner's syndrome, palatal paralysis and ataxia. Sensory loss is dissociated with ipsilateral loss of pain and temperature sensation in the face and contralateral loss in the limbs. Contralateral hemiplegia may occur if the entire half of the medulla is affected but should not be considered a feature of this discrete syndrome. Cranial nerve nuclei concerned with eye movement lie within the pons and midbrain.

18 A B E

In rheumatic fever, carditis is suggested by the presence of diastolic or long systolic murmurs, by pericarditis and by cardiomegaly (pericardial effusion excluded by echocardiography). A prolonged PR interval is very common in rheumatic fever (80%) and is present equally in those with and without carditis. Sinus arrhythmia is a normal finding.

19 A B D

Thiazide diuretics are associated with a risk of developing diabetes. The effect is dose related being more likely with bendrofluazide in a dose of 5–10 mg daily. The low dose of 2.5 mg daily has little effect on glucose tolerance and the very low dose of 1.25 mg has no effect. Corticosteroids such as prednisolone increase blood glucose, especially if high doses are used for a prolonged period. Oestrogens are associated with impaired glucose tolerance but development of diabetes is very unlikely.

20 A B D

Ciprofloxacin has good broad spectrum bactericidal and antituberculous activity. It is however inactive against anaerobes and has only moderate activity against certain Gram-positive organisms including the pneumococcus. Because of widespread drug resistance it is now the treatment of choice for typhoid fever.

21 B

The characteristic finding in thyroid eye disease is inflammatory swelling of the extraocular muscles. This impairs eye movements and subsequent fibrotic tethering may make ophthalmoplegia permanent. Inferior rectus is most commonly affected, leading to impairment of upward gaze in the abducted eye. The disease is both more severe and more common in males and cigarette smokers. Radioactive iodine has been associated with deterioration of the condition. Steroids are generally reserved for rapidly progressive disease where there is reduction in visual acuity due to optic nerve compression at the apex of the orbit.

22 A C D

Howell-Jolly bodies represent blood cells which are usually removed in the spleen and their appearance in the blood film is in keeping with splenic atrophy. Oral aphthous ulceration and osteoporosis are recognised although atypical presenting features of gluten sensitivity. Focal biliary cirrhosis is the pathognomic liver lesion in cystic fibrosis.

23 A D E

Anaphylaxis is an example of a type I reaction responsible for immediate hypersensitivity. Binding of monomeric IgE alone to the antigen has no effect but binding monomeric IgE which is cell-associated cross links immunoglobulin molecules, triggering off a series of events within the cell. Clinically these are characterized by vasodilation, bronchospasm, oedema and collection of eosinophils. It may be acquired by passive administration of antibody within 6 hours after injection. Typical type I reactions may be organ specific as in asthma or atopic dermatitis. Generalised anaphylaxis may occur if the antigen is widely distributed, manifest by marked vasodilation, oedema and shock

24 B C

Apoprotein A1 is an apolipoprotein that is predominantly associated with HDL and is representative of HDL particle number. It is inversely related to cardiovascular disease risk. It is involved in removal of cholesterol by HDL from the tissues and facilitates transfer back to VLDL and the liver. It is not involved in intestinal transport and not present in chylomicrons. It is elevated in nephrotic syndrome, along with increased HDL particle number.

25 B E

One-third of patients with idiopathic membranous glomerulonephritis (GN) progress to end-stage renal failure. The condition may recur in renal transplants, but less frequently than focal segmental glomerulosclerosis, IgA nephropathy and mesangiocapillary glomerulonephritis. Although an immune aetiology is established, circulating immune complexes do not play a major role. Secondary membranous GN is linked to solid malignancies (breast, stomach, colon) and non-Hodgkin's lymphoma; Hodgkin's disease is associated with minimal change GN. Gold and penicillamine therapy in rheumatoid arthritis may also induce a reversible secondary membranous GN.

26 D

Most (85%) insomnias are secondary to psychological factors, psychiatric or physical illness or drug-induced states; caffeine abuse is often associated. Alcohol decreases total sleep time but decreases the time required to fall asleep. Neuroleptics cause akathisia. Unlike narcolepsy, hypersomnia is not associated with an irresistible urge to sleep but consists of 'hangover' symptoms caused by excessive sleep, which leads to the need for more sleep.

27 A D E

Rheumatoid nodules, up to 1 cm in diameter, may appear in the lung. Very large nodules may be associated with coal worker's pneumoconiosis (Caplan's syndrome). Systemic sclerosis gives rise to pulmonary fibrosis and inhalation pneumonia. Pulmonary manifestations of SLE include recurrent infections, pleural effusions, atelectasis and shrinking lung syndrome.

28 C D

The gene is localized on the distal end of the short arm of chromosome 4. The precise gene abnormality is a trinucleotide repeat (CAG). Huntington's disease is associated with a subcortical dementia and early psychiatric disturbance. L-dopa medication increases chorea in symptomatic patients and has been used as a provocative test for 'at-risk' individuals.

29 A C E

Haemarthrosis occurs in Christmas disease (haemophilia B due to deficiency of factor IX). Locomotor symptoms are common in sickle cell disease but haemarthrosis does not occur. A low platelet count does not lead to haemarthrosis. Charcot joints may be affected by haemarthrosis as may pyrophosphate arthritis, probably as a consequence of inflammation.

30 B C E

The predominant influence on prolactin secretion is an inhibitory one through dopamine secretion by the hypothalamus and transport of this through the pituitary portal vessels. Clozapine is a modern antipsychotic which like all centrally acting antidopaminergic agents may inhibit the action of dopamine. Growth hormone secreting tumours may also secrete prolactin or cause hyperprolactinaemia through pituitary stalk disruption. True seizures *may* be distinguished from pseudoseizures by the elevation of prolactin which occurs in the former. Hypothyroidism (but not thyrotoxicosis) may lead to elevated serum prolactin as a consequence of reflex increase in thyrotrophin releasing hormone which has a weak prolactin stimulating effect.

31 C D E
Although there is severe hypertriglyceridaemia, WHO type 1 disease is not associated with increased ischaemic heart disease risk. HDL cholesterol (reverse cholesterol transport) values above 1.1 mmol/l appear to be protective. In angiographic studies, LDL cholesterol values below 3.4 mmol/l seem to be associated with atheroma regression and values above 4.1 mmol/l with progression. Familial hypercholesterolaemia is an autosomal dominant condition with affected heterozygotes expressing defective hepatic LDL receptors (hence reduced LDL clearance from plasma). Proteinuria and microalbuminuria are markers for later development of atheromatous disease in NIDDM.

32 A B C
Oesophageal spasm occurs in all ages and can mimic angina closely even to the extent of being relieved by GTN. The diagnosis is suggested by a corkscrew oesophagus on barium swallow and simultaneous non-peristaltic contractions on manometry.

33 B C
A lesion of the third cranial nerve causes an efferent pupillary defect, mydriasis and divergent strabismus. A midbrain lesion may produce a third cranial nerve palsy and contralateral hemiplegia (Weber's syndrome).

34 A B D E
The principal differential diagnosis is from epilepsy, which is usually characterized by a preceding aura and prolonged unconsciousness and recovery. Owing to cerebral hypoxia, tonic/clonic seizures may occur with cardiac syncope. Tachyarrhythmias (ventricular and supraventricular) may profoundly reduce cardiac output due to the sheer rapidity or by further compromising myocardial perfusion. Ventricular tachycardia may be an 'escape' rhythm precipitated by a primary bradyarrhythmia.

35 A D E

Animal bites in rabies endemic countries should be treated by thorough washing followed by rabies specific immunoglobulin and vaccination. No immune response is detectable in man and symptomatic infection is invariably fatal. The diagnosis can be confirmed by detecting rabies antigen in the dermal nerves of a full thickness skin punch biopsy taken from the hairy part of the neck.

36 A B C D E

Neurofibromatosis (Von Recklinghausen's disease) is inherited as an autosomal dominant trait. It is also associated with cutaneous fibromata and neurofibromata which may undergo sarcomatous change. Retinal phacoma also occur in tuberous sclerosis. 'Plexiform neuroma' is the term applied to diffuse neurofibromatosis of nerve trunks.

37 B C E

Precipitating antibodies against sugar cane occur in bagassosis and similar antibodies are present in histoplasmosis and bird fancier's lung. In fibrosing alveolitis, rheumatoid factor (50%), anti-nuclear factor and other non-organ specific antibodies (30%) may be present. Antibodies have not been found in byssinosis.

38 C D E

The serum ferritin and serum iron levels fall while that of transferrin rises due to increased hepatic synthesis. The anaemia, seen as a result of iron deficiency, is primarily due to defective haem synthesis. Glossitis and less commonly partial villous atrophy have been described in patients with iron deficiency and are believed to result from a reduction in iron-containing enzymes normally responsible for the maintenance of epithelial surfaces. Chronic intravascular haemolysis, such as occurs in PNH, can lead to excessive loss of iron in the urine.

39 A B C D

Hypothermia is defined as a core temperature of 35°C or less. Shivering is usually present until the temperature falls below about 30°C. Myotonia or impaired muscle relaxation is a recognized manifestation. Pancreatitis but not hepatic necrosis commonly complicates the condition. Hypothermia also impairs tissue oxygen delivery through its effect on haemoglobin-oxygen dissociation.

40 A B D E

Tetracycline use is limited by adverse effects and development of resistance by many common pathogens. Tetracycline inhibits protein synthesis and results in increased production of urea and other nitrogenous end-products. These products and tetracycline itself accumulate in the presence of poor renal function. Tetracycline binds to calcium and stains teeth during development. It should therefore be avoided during pregnancy and in children under 8 years old.

41 A C D

Anaemia in CRF is largely due to lack of erythropoietin, is least marked in polycystic renal disease, and is only consistently reversed by successful renal transplantation. The degree of anaemia is broadly related to the serum creatinine, becoming manifest when the GFR falls below 30 ml/min. Increased red cell 2,3 DPG shifts the oxygen dissociation curve to the right, increasing tissue oxygenation. Iron utilisation is disordered in CRF and iron deficiency is recognised by lack of stainable iron in the bone marrow or by a low serum ferritin.

42 B D

Insulin resistance is a feature of NIDDM, obesity and hypertension. There is associated hyperinsulinaemia, hypertriglyceridaemia and reduced HDL cholesterol. The defect is thought to be post-receptor and can be improved by physical training. Acanthosis nigricans is a cutaneous marker of insulin resistance, occurring in patients with obesity, polycystic ovary syndrome and acromegaly (it is also associated with internal malignancy).

43 A B C

Amiodarone and nifedipine displace digoxin from plasma binding protein, and quinidine and nifedipine reduce renal clearance of digoxin. Cholestyramine binds digoxin, and rifampicin induces hepatic metabolism.

44 B C E

Bioavailability after oral administration depends on drug absorption from the gut and first-pass metabolism in the bowel wall and liver. First-pass metabolism is reduced in hepatic cirrhosis, resulting in increased bioavailability. Drugs with high first-pass metabolism therefore have increased bioavailability in the presence of cirrhosis. Examples are lipid soluble beta-blockers (e.g. propranolol), most opioids, metoclopramide, most tricyclic antidepressants, lignocaine, and natural oestrogens.

45 A B D

Clinical features of acromegaly include bitemporal hemianopia due to chiasmal compression, frontal sinus hypertrophy and nerve entrapment due to soft tissue overgrowth. Biochemically, there is elevated growth hormone secretion which fails to suppress in a glucose tolerance test and elevation of insulin-like growth factor 1, which is secreted by the liver in response to growth hormone. Untreated acromegaly shortens life expectancy, largely as a consequence of cardiovascular disease but there is also an increased incidence of malignancy.

46 A B E

As with other myeloproliferative disorders with a raised granulocyte count, a raised transcobalamin I results in an elevation in serum vitamin B12. In up to 20% of all acute transformations seen in CML the blast cells demonstrate a lymphoid phenotype. Lymphadenopathy is uncommon in the early stages of CML but can be seen as the disease progresses. The Philadelphia chromosome involves a translocation between chromosomes 9 and 22. Alpha interferon can result in both complete haematological and cytogenetic remission in a minority of patients with CML.

47 A B C D

All helminths that migrate through the lungs can cause transient pulmonary symptoms. Tropical pulmonary eosinophilia is generally caused by filarial species. *Paragonimus westermani* is a lung fluke causing cavitating lesions that may be mistaken for tuberculosis. *Ancylostoma braziliensis* is a dog hookworm that causes cutaneous larva migrans in man.

48 A B C D

Osteopenia is defined as reduced bone mineral content, as assessed by quantitative radiological techniques: osteoporosis implies the presence of fractures as well. Factors which increase the risk of osteopenia and which may increase the risk of fracture include low weight, oestrogen deficiency (and testosterone deficiency in men), smoking, thyrotoxicosis, primary hyperparathyroidism, corticosteroid treatment and Cushing's syndrome, chronic liver disease, alcohol excess, immobility and transplant recipients. Reflex sympathetic dystrophy (Sudeck's atrophy or algodystrophy) is characterized by osteopenia, sweating and pain, usually following fracture.

49 A B E

In the arm, spasticity in a patient with hemiplegia is most pronounced in the flexor muscles and weakness in the extensor muscles. The converse is true in the leg. The peroneal nerve supplies skin over the lateral aspect of the lower leg. The saphenous branch of the femoral nerve supplies skin over the medial aspect of the lower leg. A sciatic nerve palsy causes weakness of hip extension, knee flexion and foot dorsiflexion, plantar flexion, inversion and eversion. A femoral nerve palsy causes weakness of knee extension.

50 A D E

OSA is seldom seen prior to middle age and daytime sleepiness is the main symptom. Sedatives, and especially alcohol, should be avoided completely if possible.

51 A B D

The most common side effect is cough which may be dose dependent. The cough is dry and may require the drugs to be stopped. Acute renal failure is a serious problem but is usually reversible if it is recognized early and the drug stopped. It is thus essential to monitor renal function.

52 A D E

The sickled red cells can result in stasis of blood in the penile tissue causing priapism; this can lead to impotence unless treated effectively. Stasis in the renal medulla can cause papillary necrosis, haematuria and even nephrogenic diabetes insipidus. The cumulative effect of multiple infarcts in the spleen commonly results in hyposplenism. The 'sickle chest syndrome' can produce symptoms consistent with those of a pneumothorax although the pathology is different. Patients with sickle cell disease can develop proliferative retinopathy, especially if haemoglobin C is also present (haemoglobin SC disease).

53 B E

Parkinson's disease is typically associated with bradykinesia, cogwheel or 'lead pipe' rigidity and resting tremor. The voice may be monotonous and hypophonic. Upward gaze is typically restricted. Supranuclear gaze palsy, pseudobulbar palsy and axial rigidity are characteristic of Steele-Richardson-Olszewski syndrome, a condition which may superficially mimic Parkinson's disease.

54 A C D

Not all inhaled inorganic dusts cause fibrosis of the lung. It is not a feature of simple coal miner's pneumoconiosis, siderosis from pure iron oxide inhalation (e.g. in welding) or stannosis (in tin smelting workers). Silica, tungsten carbide and aluminium are fibrogenic dusts.

55 A B C E
The development of tall R waves in the anterior chest leads in posterior infarction can be considered the 'mirror image' of Q waves looked at from the other side of the heart. Tricuspid atresia is associated with a very small right ventricle producing little voltage. WPW syndrome type A is associated with a tall R wave in lead V1 but type B is not.

56 B D E
Ulcerative colitis classically involves the colon and rectum causing mucosal ulceration which, if severe enough, has a pseudopolypoid appearance. It represents islands of remaining mucosa. Diarrhoea and rectal bleeding are classical presenting symptoms. Fistula formation is more typical of Crohn's disease and cobblestoning describes the X-ray appearance of the mucosa in that disease.

57 None true
Rose spots classically occur over the upper abdomen and lower thorax. They are erythematous macules that blanch on pressure and last only 3–4 days. The rash is more common in paratyphoid.

58 E
In the ISIS-2 study, intravenous streptokinase given alone within 12 hours reduced mortality by 25% at 35 days and this benefit increased to 42% when aspirin was added. Alteplase given as an accelerated regime with heparin is more effective than streptokinase alone in patients with anterior infarcts (GUSTO). Streptokinase prolongs the APTT. Efficacy is reduced by neutralizing antibodies which may be a result of recent streptococcal infection or recent administration of streptokinase. Hypertension is a contraindication as it increases the risk of haemorrhagic complications, particularly stroke.

59 B C E
Alport's syndrome is usually inherited dominantly or as X-linked recessive, whereas nephrogenic DI is an X-linked recessive condition. Patients with cystinuria have a tendency to form semi-opaque renal calculi, due to a failure of reabsorption of filtered dibasic amino acids. Cystinosis is a more severe condition in which cystine accumulates within lysosomes, leading to major pathology in kidneys, heart, eyes and blood vessels.

60 A B C D
Bronchial carcinoma is now the most common malignant disease in western Europe. Occupational risk factors include exposure to asbestos, nickel, arsenic, haematite, chromates and coal/radioactive gases.

ANSWERS TO PRACTICE EXAM 2

1   B C

Hepatocellular carcinoma is more common in men and associated with cirrhosis of any cause, the most common worldwide being hepatitis B. It is a very vascular tumour and liver biopsy is therefore relatively contraindicated. The appropriate clinical setting together with a positive ultrasound or CT scan with high serum titre of alpha fetoprotein usually suffice to make the diagnosis.

2   B C E

Neurological presentation is rare except in thrombotic thrombocytopenic purpura. Fibrin deposition produces fragmentation and platelet consumption. Heparin frequently exacerbates the bleeding tendency with fatal results.

3   A C E

Scleritis in rheumatoid disease can lead to thinning of the cornea and subsequent perforation, so called scleromalacia perforans. Conjunctivitis may occur in lupus but scleritis is not seen. Scleritis is a typical feature of Wegener's granulomatosis. Iritis is prominent in ankylosing spondylitis and scleritis does not occur.

4   A E

Motor neuropathy affecting the foot may cause deformity of the toes as a result of unopposed action of long extensor muscles, thus increasing pressure over the metatarsal area. An insensitive foot due to sensory neuropathy is clearly important and sympathetic denervation also contributes by making the skin dry, prone to callus and cracking. Thick callus increases the likelihood of ischaemic necrosis in the deeper layers of the skin and subsequent ulceration. Background retinopathy may be associated with foot ulceration but is not causally related. Blindness due to other forms of retinopathy is an important predisposing factor for ulceration. Appropriate treatment and good glycaemic control delays or prevents the development of microvascular complications.

5   A C D

Complex partial seizures of temporal lobe onset may be accompanied by an aura of fear, dread, visceral sensation and dysmnesic phenomena such as jamais vu and deja vu. Primitive visual aura suggests an occipital focus. Versive seizures with turning of the eyes and/or head to the contralateral side suggests a frontal focus.

6   A B C D E

A third heart sound (prodiastolic gallop) and mural thrombus are common in congestive cardiomyopathy. Alcoholic cardiomyopathy may respond clinically to thiamine, but withdrawal of alcohol is just as important. Dysrhythmias may be difficult to treat. Beta-blockers must be used very cautiously since they can precipitate severe pulmonary oedema and cardiogenic shock. The risk of sudden death is related to ventricular arrhythmias.

7   A D E

ACE inhibitors, such as captopril, may cause renal failure. The risk is increased in the presence of renal artery stenosis, peripheral vascular disease and cardiac failure. Renal function must be regularly monitored. Gentamicin is a well-recognized cause of renal failure. The risk is reduced by once daily dosing. NSAIDs are among the most common drugs to impair renal function, especially in elderly patients.

8   A C

Pneumococcal vaccine is a polyvalent vaccine made up of capsular polysaccharide from 23 capsular types of pneumococcus. Vaccination should be considered for all those in whom pneumococcal infection is more common and/or more serious. This includes patients with homozygous sickle cell disease, asplenia and chronic renal, cardiac, liver or respiratory disease. In HIV-positive patients serological response to vaccination, and hence benefit, decline with increasing immunocompromise. Routine revaccination is not normally recommended.

9   B C E

Both pregnancy and oral oestrogen administration lead to increased secretion of thyroxine binding globulin, with a consequent rise in total serum thyroxine concentration. Phenytoin and salicylate displace thyroxine from its plasma binding sites but negative feedback ensures that free thyroxine levels remain normal. Phenytoin may additionally lower thyroxine levels by inducing hepatic metabolism. In panhypopituitarism, the thyroid is usually affected last but by definition, there must be TSH deficiency (normal sequence of pituitary hormone loss GH, LH, FSH, ACTH, TSH).

10   B D E

Bile salt depletion may lead to gallstone formation either as a result of Crohn's disease of the terminal ileum, or following ileal resection for this condition. The unconjugated hyperbilirubinaemia of Gilbert's syndrome does not lead to gallstone formation as it is a manifestation of a failure of transport of bilirubin.

11   A B C D E
Inherited deficiencies of all 11 classical pathway proteins have been described with deficiency in several control proteins. With the exception of C1 they are all inherited as co-dominant. There are three general patterns of clinical manifestation associated with complement deficiencies: 1) connective tissue disorders with C2 deficiency; 2) recurrent pyogenic infections with C3 deficiency; and 3) recurrent sepsis with mycelia species in patients with deficiencies C5, C6, C7, C8 and C9. The genes for all complement proteins are located in the major histocompatibility complex region of chromosome 6.

12   A D
Tumour necrosis factor is a proinflammatory cytokine released primarily from macrophages in response to bacterial toxins, inflammatory products and other invasive stimuli. It is present in the circulation in free form and complexed to binding proteins derived from cleavage fragments of TNF receptors. The cellular effects of TNF include cytotoxicity against tumour cells, suppression of adipocyte lipoprotein lipase and reduction of myocyte resting membrane potential. Acute exposure to high doses of TNF causes shock, fever, vascular leak syndrome and widespread tissue injury. At low doses chronic exposure leads to cachexia and protein catabolism but tachyphylaxis to TNF actions occur.

13   A B C D
Significant cardiovascular events occur at least 20 times more frequently in dialysis patients than in the general population; cardiac arrest due to hyperkalaemia, transient systemic vasodilation and coronary disease is also well recognized during haemodialysis. Haemodialysis with cuprophane allows accumulation of beta-2-microglobulin, and development of dialysis-related amyloid. Aluminium toxicity, once common with aluminium-containing phosphate binders and with previously untreated water, is now rare due to reverse osmosis water treatment and frequent assessment of aluminium concentration.

14   A E
Many physical symptoms are associated with anxiety states: dyspnoea, difficulty inhaling, overbreathing, dry mouth, difficulty swallowing, palpitations, chest pain, frequency and urgency of micturition, tinnitus, blurred vision, paraesthesia, dizziness and sweating. Difficulty concen-

trating and complaints of poor memory occur. Persistent and objective memory loss is not present and raises the possibility of an organic cause. Depressive illnesses may present with anxiety symptoms; low mood and early morning wakening would be indicative of this. Problems getting to sleep are more usual with anxiety disorders.

15 A B C D

An apical lung tumour can invade the ipsilateral sympathetic fibres (Horner's syndrome), eighth cervical and first thoracic ventral rami (pain in fourth and fifth digits: paralysis of forearm and hand muscles) and the first rib.

16 B C D E

Myotonia is typically relieved by exercise and exacerbated by cold. Myotonia congenita can be dominantly (Thomsen's) or recessively (Becker's) inherited. Thomsen's myotonia congenita is associated with muscle hypertrophy. Myotonic dystrophy (autosomal dominant) can be distinguished by the occurrence of cataracts, ptosis, muscle wasting, gonadal atrophy and cardiomyopathy. The EMG invariably shows typical myotonic (dive bomber) discharges.

17 A C D E

The core clinical features are severe and prolonged pain which is inconsistent with anatomical patterns of innervation, and the absence of an organic cause. Patients have usually been extensively investigated. The onset of pain may be related to emotionally difficult events. The pain may allow the patient to avoid certain activities and result in attention from relatives and friends. However the patient does not intentionally produce the pain. The pain may be associated with a depressive illness, and may respond to antidepressants (response may also occur in the absence of overt depression). Response to standard analgesics is poor. The course of psychogenic pain is variable and may persist for years.

18 A C E

Glucagon is secreted by the pancreas in response to hypoglycaemia. It elevates blood glucose by increasing hepatic glucose production through gluconeogenesis and glycogenolysis, both actions being mediated by cyclic AMP. Paradoxically, glucagon stimulates insulin secretion. Its positive inotropic action has been exploited occasionally in the treatment of severe beta blocker poisoning.

19 A B D

By inhibiting the synthesis of cholesterol in the liver from acetate, HMG CoA reductase inhibitors (statins) reduce hepatic secretion of LDL cholesterol. Cholestyramine binds bile acids in the gut, preventing their reabsorption and encouraging the synthesis of new bile acids from hepatic cholesterol. All fibrates reduce LDL cholesterol by a variety of mechanisms and also reduce plasma triglyceride. Marine oils lower triglyceride concentrations and may exacerbate hypercholesterolaemia. Propranolol produces a small rise in LDL cholesterol and a small fall in HDL cholesterol.

20 E

Octreotide increases small intestinal transit time; it is given subcutaneously to control high stoma output. It has only limited direct effect on portal veins and reduces portal venous pressure predominantly by reducing splanchnic arterial blood flow.

21 C

The posterior interosseous nerve (C6,7,8) is a branch of the radial nerve (C5,6,7,8). The brachioradialis is supplied by the radial nerve proximal to the posterior interosseous nerve branch. Flexor pollicis longus is supplied by the anterior interosseous nerve (C7,8). Opponens pollicis is supplied by the median nerve (C6,7,8,T1).

22 A B C D E

Mitral annular calcification is an independent risk factor for embolic stroke (relative risk x2), as is atrial fibrillation in non-rheumatic (x6) and rheumatic (x17) heart disease. Coarctation of the aorta is associated with upper body hypertension and berry aneurysms, which predispose to intracranial haemorrhage. Rarely, a patent foramen ovale may allow passage of a paradoxical embolus (i.e. from right to left atrium).

23 A D E

Symptomatic meningitis occurs in 5–10% of patients but it is usually mild. CSF abnormalities (lymphocytosis and virus isolation) are more common. Pancreatitis is very rare and the amylase may be raised due to parotitis. Oophoritis is a well known complication and like orchitis is nearly always unilateral.

24 B C E

Demyelination typically affects white matter of the brain and spinal cord. It may occasionally affect grey matter of the cerebral cortex but only rarely affects the grey matter of the spinal cord.

25 A C D E

Extrinsic allergic alveolitis characteristically produces a high lymphocyte percentage consisting of T8 suppressor cells in contrast to sarcoid in which T4 helper cells predominate. A normal lavage consists of 90% alveolar macrophages, 10% lymphocytes and 1% neutrophils.

26 A C D

Sideroblastic anaemia is associated with a hypochromic anaemia that may be either macrocytic or microcytic depending on the underlying cause. In cases of acute haemorrhage that occur prior to the development of iron deficiency the blood film may appear normochromic/normocytic if examined before the onset of a reticulocyte response (2–3 days). Long-term treatment with phenytoin can be followed by folate deficiency. Possible mechanisms include inhibition of absorbtion, inhibition of folate-dependent enzymes and induction of folate-utilizing enzymes.

27 A C

The relatively recently described CA125 antigen is a useful tumour marker in some forms of ovarian carcinoma. Alpha fetoprotein levels are increased with both hepatoma and malignant teratoma. Embryonic tumours may also secrete HCG, as in choriocarcinoma and teratoma. Medullary carcinoma of the thyroid characteristically produces calcitonin: thyroglobulin may however be a useful tumour marker for other thyroid cell carcinomas. PTH related peptide is the main mediator of the humoral hypercalcaemia of malignancy and is most commonly produced by tumours of epithelial rather than mesenchymal origin.

28 D E

Metoclopramide is an antagonist at D2 dopamine receptors. It increases the rate of gastric emptying. Extrapyramidal reactions are particularly common in children and young adults. Metoclopramide increases prolactin release and thus may cause galactorrhoea.

29 A B C E

Renal failure in myeloma is characteristically associated with eosinophilic intratubular casts in the distal part of the nephron associated with a giant cell reaction. Chronic renal failure may also complicate renal amyloidosis, which occurs in about 10% of cases. Glomerular abnormalities are, however, usually minor. Acute renal failure may follow intravenous pyelography due to precipitation of light chains during dehydration. Hypercalcaemia may precipitate renal failure and if reversed may result in improvement in renal function. Uric acid crystal nephropathy can be avoided by the use of allopurinol.

30 A C E

p53 is a tumour suppressor gene present on chromosome 17. It is not a viral protein. It encodes a nuclear phosphoprotein that acts as a transcription factor; it delays entry into S phase of the cell division cycle thus allowing time for DNA repair to occur before cell replication. Mutation of p53 promotes tumour formation. Somatic mutation of the p53 gene occurs at both alleles in 50–80% of spontaneous human cancers. p53 is not required for normal development, but is a necessary cofactor for programmed cell death (apoptosis).

31 B E

These drugs inhibit calcium influx during stage 2. The negatively inotropic effect of verapamil may be fatal if given to a patient in VT.

32 A C D E

Enzyme induction may occur with several drugs and hydrocarbons. There is an increase in the activity of the enzymes which metabolise drugs and natural compounds. Osteomalacia may occur because of increased breakdown of vitamin D metabolites. Low dose oestrogen pills may be metabolised too quickly such that the lower plasma concentrations fail to inhibit ovulation. Smoking increases the activity of liver enzymes other than those induced by most drugs. Bilirubin conjugation is increased by enzyme induction with a resulting fall in plasma concentration.

33 A B C D

The karyotype in Klinefelter's syndrome is characterized by one or more extra X chromosomes. The IQ and other features of disease severity are usually related to the number of X chromosomes. Patients are usually tall, long limbed, with very small testes, gynaecomastia and primary infertility due to azoospermia. FSH and LH are normally both elevated. Characteristically, they retain a good head of hair and are not prone to balding, which is androgen dependent.

34 D E

AIHA is seen as a complication of lymphoproliferative disorders such as chronic lymphocytic leukaemia, Hodgkin's and non-Hodgkin's lymphoma. Rarely the disorder can be mediated via classes of immunoglobulin other than IgG such as IgM and IgA and in some instances the direct antiglobulin test can be negative. The AIHA seen following infection with *Mycoplasma pneumoniae* is of the cold-type. The classic example of drug-induced warm AIHA occurs following administration of methyldopa but other drugs, including L-dopa, have been associated with the disorder.

35 B D E

Schistosoma mansoni is principally found in Africa and South America. Chronic disease mainly affects the gut and liver although the brain, spinal cord and lungs may also be affected. Praziquantel and oxamniquine are the two main choices in treatment. Cercarial dermatitis (swimmer's itch) may follow exposure to water containing any schistosomes.

36 A B C

Magnesium is lost from the extracellular fluid in diabetic ketoacidosis and diarrhoea. Hypomagnesaemia may also follow long term use of loop diuretics. Magnesium is predominantly an intracellular ion and behaves in this respect like potassium. However, extracellular magnesium is predominantly protein bound and is handled in a similar way to calcium. Magnesium has been used to prevent ventricular arrhythmias but hypomagnesaemia is not a direct consequence of acute myocardial infarction.

37 A C D

All calcium channel blockers have some negative inotropic action but this is minimal for some of the dihydropyridine derivatives. Verapamil has most negative inotropic and A–V blocking action and diltiazem has intermediate effects. Lisinopril has beneficial effects on cardiac function without intrinsic negative inotropic action. Propafenone, an antiarrhythmic agent has significant negative inotropic effect and weak beta adrenoceptor blocking action. Bisoprolol is a highly selective beta-1 adrenoceptor antagonist. Thyroxine increases myocardial contractility and oxygen consumption in hypothyroid patients.

38 A B D

Drugs which may produce pulmonary fibrosis include amiodarone, busulphan, melphalan, cyclophosphamide and bleomycin. Pulmonary oedema may occur as an adverse reaction to hydrochlorothiazide, phenylbutazone, beta-2-agonists and bleomycins. Barbiturates may produce profound respiratory depression. Phenytoin is one of a number of drugs which have been associated with a lupus like syndrome; others include hydrallazine, procainamide and isoniazid. Prostaglandin F2 alpha is a potent bronchoconstrictor and prostaglandin E2 is a bronchodilator although this has yet to be exploited therapeutically.

39 A C E

Parkinson-like effects are brought about by dopaminergic deficit in the nigrostriatal tracts. Drugs which antagonise the action of dopamine at receptors in this area and thus produce the effects, are the neuroleptics, haloperidol, prochlorperazine and trifluoperazine. Imipramine is a central muscarinic antagonist of acetylcholine and phenytoin is likewise without action at dopamine receptors.

40 A B D

Approximately 10–15% of patients with myeloma have Bence-Jones proteinuria in the absence of a serum paraprotein. Infiltration of the bone marrow from any cause can result in a leucoerythroblastic blood picture. Up to 60% of patients with myeloma present with symptoms of bone pain. Amyloid can occur as a complication of myeloma and cause compression of the median nerve in the carpal tunnel. The incidence of myeloma rises with age, the median age at presentation is 70 years and only 2% of patients are below 40 years of age.

41 None true

Ranitidine is a competitive inhibitor of histamine H2 receptors. The prokinetic effects of cisapride are mediated through cholinergic stimulation and the actions of domperidone are related to blockade of dopamine receptors. Omeprazole inhibits gastric acid secretion and leads to a rise in intragastric pH. Sucralfate is an aluminium based mucoprotective agent with only weak acid neutralising properties.

42 D

Prednisolone is as effective as hydrocortisone given normal absorption. Bacterial infections are uncommon in acute asthma and therefore antibiotics are not indicated routinely. A high or rising pCO_2 is one of the indications for ventilation.

43 A C D E

The deficiency of vitamin B12 results in a failure to transport folate from the plasma to intracellular sites. Antibodies to intrinsic factor are found in the serum of approximately half of all patients with PA; they are present in the gastric juice of 80% of patients. The pathophysiology is essentially that of an autoimmune disorder leading to gastric atrophy. Although therapy with corticosteroids improves the gastric lesion with a return of secretion of intrinsic factor the disease is best managed by life-long vitamin B12 supplements.

44 A C D E

A third heart sound reflects rapid ventricular filling in early diastole and may be a consequence of ventricular decompensation or A–V valve regurgitation. Significant mitral stenosis prevents rapid left ventricular filling but beware, a right-sided third heart sound may co-exist with mitral stenosis. In constrictive pericarditis the restrictive effect of the adherent pericardium halts diastolic filling abruptly, producing a third heart sound (pericardial knock).

45 B D E

Creutzfeldt-Jakob disease is a transmissible spongiform encephalopathy which is thought to be due to an abnormal prion protein (PrP). It is rapidly progressive with death usually within 12–18 months of onset. The EEG is markedly abnormal with repetitive triphasic discharges on a flat background.

46 A C

The membrane attack complex (C5b-9) assembles following cleavage of C5 to form C5b via the classical or alternative pathway. It inserts into cell membranes resulting in a transmembrane channel that leads to cell lysis. Its binding to cells is inhibited by VLDL and autologous cells contain membrane control proteins that partially protect them from the action of MAC. Hereditary angioneurotic oedema is caused by C1 esterase inhibitor deficiency allowing excessive C1 activity. PNH is caused by reduced membrane control proteins resulting in increased sensitivity to MAC.

47 A C

Pleural plaques only indicate asbestos exposure and are not pre-malignant. Diffuse fibrosis, not pulmonary nodules are found, and bronchial carcinoma is a recognized complication of pulmonary involvement.

48 B E

Normal pressure hydrocephalus is associated with the clinical triad of subcortical dementia, gait disturbance and urinary incontinence. The gait disturbance is usually postural and broad based. The term 'gait apraxia' has been applied but it is not due to primary cerebral cortical dysfunction. The lateral ventricles are enlarged, resulting in greater deviation of fibres from the medial cerebral cortex (leg and sphincter motor fibres). CSF pressure studies demonstrate an intermittent rise in CSF pressure. Good prognostic factors for improvement following a CSF shunting procedure are: known aetiology (e.g. subarachnoid haemorrhage), short duration of symptoms, motor signs and transient improvement following CSF drainage (lumbar puncture).

49   A D E

The MHC (major histocompatibility complex) on chromosome 6 encodes the polymorphic cell surface glycoproteins of the HLA (human leucocyte antigen) system. Class I molecules (HLA-A, B and C) are associated with beta-2-microglobulin and are constitutively expressed on most cells. Class II molecules (HLA-DP, DQ and DR) are constitutively expressed only on a few cell types (B lymphocytes, macrophages, monocytes and follicular dendritic cells) but can be induced by interferon in a wide variety of tissues (including endothelial cells, pancreatic beta cells and renal tubular cells) and present antigen to T cells.

50   B C D

A is false, many other symmetrical distributions exist. E is false, the standard error is a measure of the reliability of a mean value.

51   B C D E

The central clinical features of bulimia nervosa are an intractable urge to overeat, self induced vomiting and laxative abuse. Patients are usually of normal weight. Most patients are female and usually menstruate normally. Patients have distorted body image. Depressive symptoms are common.

52   B D

Haemophilia A (factor eight deficiency) is X-linked; haemophilia B is autosomal recessive. Congenital pyloric stenosis has no simple Mendelian pattern of inheritance; rather, it is the result of a combination of environmental and gene effects so that a sibling has an increased risk of developing the illness. Nephrogenic diabetes is X-linked recessive. Ataxia telangiectasia is autosomal recessive.

53   B C D

Prophylaxis against opportunistic infections has been the main advance in the care of HIV-positive patients. Cotrimoxazole is the drug of choice for PCP prophylaxis and also gives good prophylaxis against toxoplasma encephalitis. Rifabutin delays the onset of MACBAC but has not been shown to prolong life.

54   B C

The median nerve supplies the first and second lumbricals. The ulnar nerve (C7,8,T1) supplies the majority of the intrinsic muscles of the hand including the dorsal interossei, adductor pollicis and the third and fourth lumbricals.

55 B D E

Hair loss which is commonly asymptomatic in alopecia areata may occur at any site. Most of the follicles retain the ability to form new hairs. Alopecia areata may be associated with frank or subclinical auto-immune thyroid disease and Down's syndrome. Nail pitting or roughness is commonly found in alopecia areata.

56 A C D

Mycoplasma occurs in 3 to 4 yearly cycles. Adverse prognostic indicators include an admission serum urea greater than 7 mmol/l, diastolic blood pressure of less than 60 mm Hg and increasing age. Hypoxia is quite common in acute pneumonia but usually with a normal carbon dioxide (type I respiratory failure).

57 A B D E

Sensory disturbance is not a feature of motor neurone disease. Familial cases may exhibit extrapyramidal signs and dementia.

58 A C

Two-thirds of patients with mitral stenosis are women. Although only half of patients may give a history of rheumatic fever, the aetiology of mitral stenosis is nearly always rheumatic. Shortness of breath due to elevated left atrial pressure (increasing on exertion) is the principal symptom. The resulting elevation of pulmonary arterial pressure, to maintain pulmonary flow, frequently leads to right ventricular dysfunction. This is the usual mechanism of the tricuspid regurgitation in mitral stenosis. Rheumatic involvement of the tricuspid valve is uncommon. Some patients remain in sinus rhythm despite moderately severe mitral stenosis.

59 C

Cystic fibrosis is an autosomal recessive disease affecting 1 in 2500 live births. There is a generalised epithelial defect in chloride transport due to a variety (>300) of mutations in the CF transmembrane conductance regulator gene. The recombinant gene can be delivered to the lungs using a viral vector (or carrier) to infect the respiratory epithelium but the gene product does not incorporate into the host's genome and treatment must be repeated monthly.

60 B

Polycystic ovaries are found in up to 20% of young women but the majority do not have the syndrome associated with oligomenorrhoea, hirsutism and infertility. Patients may be obese or non-obese. Infertility is characteristically due to anovulation. Biochemical findings typically include elevated LH to FSH ratio, elevated serum testosterone, androstenedione, oestrone and a reduced concentration of sex hormone binding globulin. Hyperprolactinaemia may interfere with gonadotrophin secretion and cause anovulation but does not produce the other abnormalities. Female athletes and ballet dancers develop amenorrhoea as a consequence of low weight and hypothalamic disturbance.

ANSWERS TO PRACTICE EXAM 3

1   **A B C**
Antibodies to ds-DNA are very specific for SLE but are only seen in 60% of patients. They may be detected either by radio-immunoassay or by use of the haemoflagellate *Crithidia luciliae*. Single stranded antibodies to single stranded DNA are much less specific and are found in a very wide variety of disorders. They may have some pathogenic role. Patterns of nuclear immunofluorescence may be of some limited use. Homogenous and speckled patterns are very non-specific. The peripheral pattern is almost exclusively seen in SLE and a nucleolar pattern and centromere pattern predominantly in systemic sclerosis, the latter being associated with a CREST syndrome. Titres of antinuclear factors are not helpful in monitoring disease activity.

2   **B D E**
Antiphospholipid antibodies are associated with widespread arterial and venous thrombosis. They are a common cause of recurrent spontaneous abortion, due to placental vessel thrombosis and ischaemia. Rarely Addison's disease can result from adrenal thrombosis. Antibodies are neither specific nor sensitive for SLE but cause the laboratory phenomenon of lupus anticoagulants. The bleeding time is normal. Valvular heart disease is common in the antiphospholipid syndrome and can manifest as culture negative endocarditis.

3   **B C**
Escherichia coli accounts for three-quarters of urinary tract infections in general practice. *Proteus mirabilis* infection is common in hospital practice and points to the possibility of renal tract abnormalities, renal calculi, and previous operative intervention. Inadequate bladder emptying due to bladder neck obstruction impairs bacterial elimination, the infection arising from faecal organisms ascending from the perineum. In the absence of urinary tract abnormalities, renal calculi and analgesic abuse, urinary tract infection is rarely associated with renal failure.

4   A E

Obsessive-compulsive disorders are characterized by obsessional thinking and compulsive behaviour. Obsessional thoughts are words, ideas or beliefs that intrude into the patient's mind. They are recognized as the patient's own thoughts, are alien to their personality and are seen as nonsensical. They are usually unpleasant, are resisted and are associated with anxiety. Obsessional thoughts lead to obsessional actions which may reduce anxiety. Obsessional ruminations are endless internal debates, sometimes about insignificant details. In a minority of patients this may lead to obsessional slowness. Obsessional impulses are urges to perform acts which are often embarrassing or violent, they are seldom acted upon. Anxiety and depression are commonly associated. Men and women are equally affected. Two-thirds improve by the end of a year, cases of more than one year run a fluctuating course.

5   B D E

The right main bronchus leaves the trachea at the angle closer to the vertical than the left, and therefore the right lung is more commonly affected. Material is often aspirated into the posterior segments of the upper lobes and the apical segments of the lower lobes. The basal segments of the lower lobe are often spared as the patient is usually lying down when aspiration occurs.

6   B D E

Manganese and carbon monoxide poisoning may produce a Parkinsonian syndrome. N-methyl-4-phenyl-1,2,3,6-tetrahydropyridine (MPTP) is a synthetic opiate drug which is metabolised to the neurotoxic MPP+ to produce a Parkinsonian syndrome very similar to Parkinson's disease. In Huntington's disease of juvenile onset, extrapyramidal involvement can predominate to give a rigid-akinetic syndrome with little or no chorea.

7   A B C D

Benzodiazepines are anxiolytic, sedative, anticonvulsant and act as a muscle relaxant. They enhance GABA neurotransmission. Benzodiazepines are well tolerated and side effects tend to be a result of overdosage which leads to ataxia, drowsiness and confused thinking especially in the elderly. They potentiate the effects of central nervous system depressants such as alcohol. Dosage should be reduced in patients with impaired renal and liver function.

8   A B D

ANP is a 28 amino acid peptide secreted in response to stretching of both right and left atrial myocardium. Enlargement of the heart in congestive cardiac failure increases secretion which promotes renal sodium loss and inhibits aldosterone release.

9 B

Glibenclamide has a relatively long biological half life although it is shorter than chlorpropamide. Unfortunately, it also has biologically active metabolites with a long half life which are excreted by the kidney. This therefore precludes the use of glibenclamide in patients with renal impairment. It should be used with caution in the elderly. Gliclazide is metabolised by the liver to inactive metabolites and is therefore the sulphonylurea of choice in patients with renal impairment. Despite strong protein binding, all sulphonylureas cross the placenta, producing foetal hyperinsulinaemia and predisposing to macrosomia and neonatal hypoglycaemia. All sulphonylureas act by stimulating insulin secretion which inhibits gluconeogenesis.

10 A C D E

Erythromycin estolate causes cholestatic jaundice but other formulations of erythromycin do not. The other calcium antagonists may also rarely produce cholestasis. A number of phenothiazines and tricyclic antidepressants have been reported to produce cholestatic jaundice.

11 B

The anterior interosseous nerve is a branch of the median nerve (C6,7,8,T1). Abductor pollicis brevis and the first and second lumbricals are supplied by the median nerve. Extensor pollicis longus is supplied by the posterior interosseous nerve.

12 A C D

Occasional cannon 'a' waves occur when atrial systole is coincident with a closed mitral valve, and variability of the first heart sound relates to the timing of atrial systole in relation to mitral valve closure. Any evidence of atrial activity at the same rate as the ventricle is suggestive of association between the atria and ventricular activity. Fusion on the ECG (morphology of the QRS complex that fuses features of the VT and the sinus rhythm morphologies) occurs when there are two depolarising wavefronts within the ventricle – one from the VT focus, and one from critically timed atrial activity being able to penetrate the AV node and activate the ventricles via the His-Purkinje system. Adenosine, an AV-nodal blocker, is usually ineffective in VT.

13 B C E

Hantavirus has no arthropod vector. The reservoir of infection is in wild rodents. Nephropathia epidemica is a less severe form of haemorrhagic fever with renal syndrome and occurs primarily in Scandinavia. Recent outbreaks of Hantavirus in the USA have been associated with pulmonary disease.

14 A C E

Syringomyelic cavities typically involve the anterior aspect of the cervical and upper thoracic cord. Involvement of the spinothalamic tract produces a dissociated sensory loss in the upper limbs. The posterior columns are typically spared. Involvement of anterior horn cells produces lower motor neurone signs in the upper limbs and corticospinal tract involvement leads to upper motor neurone signs in the lower limbs. The syrinx may extend into the medulla to produce a (true) bulbar palsy (syringobulbia) and occasionally into the thoracolumbar cord. Associated anomalies at the craniovertebral junction (Arnold-Chiari malformation) can produce nystagmus.

15 A C D

Angiotensin converting enzyme inactivates bradykinin. Levels may be raised in sarcoid and also in tuberculosis, berylliosis, silicosis, asbestosis, carcinoma of the lung, primary biliary cirrhosis and leprosy. ACE inhibitors may increase ACE levels in active sarcoidosis but not in normals.

16 A C

All are causes of macrocytosis. Tropical sprue produces malabsorption. In pernicious anaemia, serum folate levels are normal or high. The megaloblastic anaemia of pregnancy or alcoholism is usually due to dietary deficiency. Lack of thyroxine, liver disease and chronic lung disease can produce macrocytosis with a normal B12 and folate level.

17 C D E

The characteristic ocular abnormality in Wilson's disease is the Kayser-Fleischer ring due to copper accumulation in the cornea. As the disease progresses, liver damage occurs and the pathological changes of chronic active hepatitis and cirrhosis become evident. Osteomalacia may follow phosphate wasting from the kidney, in turn due to copper associated tubular damage. Biochemically, there is a reduced serum caeruloplasmin (copper binding protein) and an increased urinary excretion of copper.

18 A C D E

Metformin has an antihyperglycaemic rather than a hypoglycaemic effect. It does not stimulate insulin release and does not cause hypoglycaemia.

104

Metformin is excreted unchanged by the kidney and accumulates in the presence of renal failure. Metformin may induce malabsorption of several substances, including vitamin B12.

19 D

Renal vasculitis usually involves small vessel inflammation as in microvascular polyarteritis, Wegener's and SLE; infarction is uncommon. A crescentic GN is the most common lesion, and urinary red cells and casts may point to the diagnosis. Systemic ill health with pyrexia, weight loss, myalgia and arthralgia often precede the renal presentation; eosinophilia occurs in polyarteritis nodosa and Churg-Strauss syndrome and is therefore uncommon. With prompt diagnosis and immunosuppressive therapy progression of the disease can be prevented in the majority of cases.

20 C D

Renal renin is synthesized, stored and released from the cells located in the afferent glomerular arteriole (juxtaglomerular cells). Renin acts on angiotensinogen to produce angiotensin I. The transcription rate of the renin gene is stimulated by cyclic AMP and inhibited by angiotensin II: treatment with ACE inhibitors stimulates transcription. Renin release is stimulated by lowered renal perfusion pressure, reduced delivery of chloride to the macula densa and renal nerve stimulation. However, circulating renin concentration is a poor predictor of renal artery stenosis.

21 A B C D E

The aetiology of the hypercholesterolaemia associated with anorexia is not clearly defined. Chronic renal failure, particularly where there is nephrotic syndrome may be associated with very high levels of circulating lipids. Hypothyroidism classically produces an elevation of cholesterol (type II). Therapeutic doses of steroids may produce a mixed picture and alcohol excess typically causes a high serum triglyceride level.

22 A B D

The major pathway of paracetamol metabolism is saturable. Glutathione helps to inactivate the toxic intermediate metabolite but cells are damaged as supplies become exhausted. Plasma paracetamol concentrations above a critical threshold 4–12 hours after ingestion indicate risks of liver cell damage. The first direct evidence of damage is a slow decay of paracetamol concentration or prolongation of the prothrombin time. Acetylcysteine at adequate concentration reactivates oxidised glutathione but once hepatic coma is established response to any therapy is poor.

23   A B C D E

Diabetes insipidus normally follows destruction of the posterior lobe of the pituitary or part of the hypothalamus. This may occur with space occupying or granulomatous lesions. Severe head injury may cause transient or rarely permanent cranial diabetes insipidus, probably as a consequence of damage to the pituitary stalk.

24   A B C D E

The worsening pruritus is due to histamine release. Iron deficiency is almost invariable. Gout is due to high cellular turnover. Raised leucocyte alkaline phosphatase could be due to infection or thrombosis. Splenomegaly is the only physical finding of diagnostic significance.

25   A D E

The haemolytic uraemic syndrome occurs in both enterohaemorrhagic coli and *Shigella dysenteriae* infections. Enteropathogenic strains include the subgroup of enteroadherent *E. coli* which are associated with childhood diarrhoea and probably also play an important role in chronic diarrhoea and childhood malnutrition in developing countries.

26   B C

Renal sodium loss is excessive when there is damage to the medullary tissue (as in chronic pyelonephritis) and following relief of obstruction. Severe dehydration alone, without the development of acute tubular necrosis, leads to avid conservation of sodium by the kidney, with urinary sodium concentration as low as 5 mmol/l. Once acute tubular necrosis has developed, the ability to conserve sodium correctly is lost. In cranial diabetes insipidus, the urine is very dilute, with conservation of sodium to maintain plasma volume (via activation of the renin angiotensin aldosterone axis).

27   A B

Pick's disease is a primary degenerative condition with a fronto-temporal distribution of cerebral pathology which is quite distinct from that in Alzheimer's disease. Behavioural disturbance and frontal lobe release signs are typical early clinical features. Extrapyramidal rigidity may be a late clinical feature. The EEG is usually normal. It is familial in approximately 20% of cases.

28   A B

Farmers' lung is usually caused by *Micropolyspora faeni* which flourishes in hay which has been harvested without drying. Breathlessness, rigors, fever and a dry cough occur 2–6 hours after exposure. Marked eosinophilia is not a feature.

29 C D E
Carbamazepine, phenytoin and rifampicin are potent inducers of hepatic mixed function oxidase. The clearance of the steroids is increased, the plasma concentrations fall and break-through bleeding may occur. Neither diazepam nor isoniazid induces steroid metabolism.

30 A C D E
A is true and may be complicated by DIC, and even in Hodgkin's splenectomy is currently less popular in view of A. Splenic atrophy may occur in all inflammatory bowel disorders. E is true although spherocytes remain in peripheral blood. Howell-Jolly bodies in the presence of acanthocytosis are virtually pathognomonic of reduced splenic function.

31 A B C D
Recent infarction and cardiac surgery both predispose to atrial fibrillation which is usually transient. Sinus tachycardia is typical in anxiety, while in hyperthyroidism, sinus tachycardia or atrial fibrillation may occur. Long standing hypertension is the setting in which atrial fibrillation most often occurs in the UK.

32 D
The Austin-Flint murmur may be distinguished from that caused by mitral stenosis because of the absence of a mitral opening snap. Significant compensated aortic regurgitation is usually associated with an aortic ejection murmur due to the increased stroke volume required to maintain cardiac output. As regurgitation worsens there is a tendency to a shortening of the early diastolic murmur, and a reduction of diastolic blood pressure. Antibiotic prophylaxis is indicated.

33 A B D
Elemental diet alone has been shown to be as effective at inducing remission of active Crohn's disease as steroid therapy. More recently 5-ASA compounds delivered in the appropriate form to the small intestine can also induce remission of active disease and maintain improvement.

34 B C D E
Non-metastatic manifestations of carcinoma of the bronchus include cerebellar degeneration, hypercalcaemia, ectopic ACTH production (high molecular weight forms) and hypertrophic pulmonary osteoarthropathy.

35 B C D E

Myoclonus is not a feature of Pick's disease but may be a late clinical manifestation of Alzheimer's disease. Myoclonus is a prominent and relatively early clinical feature of subacute sclerosing panencephalitis and Creutzfeldt-Jakob disease. Primary generalized epilepsy is associated with three main seizure types: generalized absence seizures (petit-mal), generalized tonic–clonic seizures (grand-mal) and myoclonic seizures. Juvenile myoclonic epilepsy is generally considered to be a sub-type of primary generalised epilepsy in which myoclonic seizures are a particularly prominent feature. Post anoxic brain damage causes myoclonus which is most marked on intention (action myoclonus).

36 B D E

Carbon dioxide is carried in the blood as bicarbonate (65%), as carbamino compounds with haemoglobin and plasma proteins (27%) and in simple solution (8%). When the saturation of haemoglobin with oxygen increases in the lungs, hydrogen ions combine with bicarbonate to produce carbonic acid which is rapidly dehydrated to give free CO_2. In conditions of impaired diffusing capacity, oxygen diffusion is affected more than CO_2 and thus in fibrosing alveolitis, hypoxia develops rather than hypercapnia.

37 B C E

Legionella pneumophila is a Gram-negative bacillus. The organism multiplies in water but infection is by inhalation. The subsequent illness varies from mild bronchitis to severe pneumonia. Pontiac fever is an acute flu like illness without pneumonia which requires symptomatic therapy only.

38 B E

A lateral medullary, dorsolateral pontine and dorsolateral midbrain lesion may produce an ipsilateral Horner's syndrome. In addition, a basal and paramedian midbrain lesion may produce an ipsilateral third cranial nerve palsy. Myotonic dystrophy may be associated with bilateral partial ptosis.

39 A B D E

Currently immunosuppressive regimes, in most transplant units, include corticosteroids. Complications attributed to steroid therapy include avascular necrosis of bone, most commonly to the hip, cataracts producing visual impairment and growth retardation. Hirsutism is a common complication of cyclosporin A therapy which is invariably a component of the immunosuppressive drug regime. There is an increased incidence of malignancy particularly malignant lymphoma and skin cancer.

40 A C E

Endothelin-1 is a 21 amino acid peptide, produced primarily from endothelial cells. It is secreted as a prohormome and endothelin-1 is generated by the action of endothelial membrane bound endothelin converting enzyme. Endothelin-1 is a potent long acting vasoconstrictor and bronchoconstrictor. Unlike angiotensin, it has equal effects on afferent and efferent glomerular arterioles. Endothelin-1 levels are elevated in acute myocardial infarction, chronic heart failure, acute renal failure, asthma and primary pulmonary hypertension.

41 B D E

A is false, two Normal distributions are best compared by use of a parametric test. C is false, Student's paired t-test requires knowledge of the mean difference between the pairs of observations.

42 B C

A hysterical symptom is one that suggests physical illness but occurs in the absence of physical disease and is not produced deliberately. Hysterical symptoms occur in association with several psychiatric disorders: depression, anxiety and organic mental disorder. 'La belle indifference' is a characteristic, but is not always present. Hysterical symptoms developing for the first time in middle or old age should raise a high suspicion of organic disease. There are usually obvious discrepancies between signs and symptoms of hysteria and those of organic disease, although this depends on the patient's medical knowledge.

43 C D E

Restriction fragment length polymorphisms are inherited variations in the size of DNA fragments produced when DNA is cut with specific (restriction) enzymes. A particular fragment size can be shown to be linked to a particular genetic disorder, generally using family studies. Oligonucleotide probes recognize the normal gene or an abnormal gene but will not detect a deletion; they are most useful for detecting point mutations (e.g. sickle cell). Gaucher's disease may be detected by demonstrating abnormal enzyme function. Haemophilia A may be diagnosed using gene probes.

44 B D E

Cryptococcus neoformans is a fungus found throughout the world. Meningitis is typically of insidious onset with headache, neck stiffness, fever, nausea and vomiting. Only 5% of patients have negative CSF cryptococcal antigen tests. Standard treatment is with intravenous amphotericin B and oral flucytosine. Relapses occur in 10–20% of patients.

45 A B

The obturator nerve (L2,3,4) supplies gracilis and adductor brevis, longus and magnus. The femoral nerve (L2,3,4) supplies quadriceps femoris. The inferior gluteal nerve (L5,S1,2) supplies gluteus maximus.

46 A C

Acute hand or foot eczema may present with a vesicular eruption known as pompholyx. Dermatitis herpetiformis is characterized by itchy vesicles arising on normal or erythematous skin, often on extensor surfaces. In exfoliative dermatitis the skin becomes reddened and then peels without blister formation. Blistering occurs in erythropoietic protoporphyria, porphyria cutanea tarda and variegate porphyria. Cutaneous sarcoidosis presents with papular or nodular eruption.

47 A C

In sarcoidosis with erythema nodosum the Kveim test is positive in 90% of patients. Bilateral hilar adenopathy is common but pulmonary symptoms are uncommon in spite of diffuse pulmonary involvement. Cardiac problems are usually due to pre-existing disease. Bone involvement and calcium metabolism are unrelated: the hypercalciuria and hypercalcaemia are a consequence of 25-hydroxylation of vitamin D in granulomatous tissue.

48 C D E

Dystrophia myotonica is an autosomal dominant disorder. The abnormal gene is a trinucleotide repeat on chromosome 19. The clinical manifestations are more pronounced in succeeding generations (anticipation), particularly if the affected parent is female. Cataracts, gonadal atrophy, cardiomyopathy and dementia may occur.

49 B C E

Paroxysmal nocturnal haemoglobinuria (PNH) is an acquired genetic disorder of the glycosyl-phosphatidylinositol anchor that binds complement neutralising proteins to red cell membranes. The result is increased red cell sensitivity to autologous complement lysis. This is exacerbated by acidosis, explaining the nocturnal nature of haemolysis and is the basis for Hams acid lysis test. PNH is associated with aplastic anaemia and a number of leukaemias.

50 B E

Physiological (pubertal) gynaecomastia is a consequence of oestrogenisation of the male breast. Gynaecomastia also occurs with a number of drugs including cimetidine and spironolactone. Diabetes mellitus is not a recognised cause but gynaecomastia may be seen in men with thyrotoxicosis, due to the elevation of plasma sex hormone binding globulin caused by the excess thyroid hormones. Oestrogen treatment and orchidectomy for prostatic carcinoma may cause gynaecomastia, but the disease itself does not.

51 A B E

Portal hypertension may result from peripancreatic fibrosis. Endoscopic retrograde pancreatography is the gold standard for making the diagnosis. Steatorrhoea results only when 90% of exocrine function is lost. The high incidence of peripheral vascular disease is not solely a reflection of the tendency to develop diabetes secondary to endocrine failure.

52 A C D

Protein C is a vitamin K dependent protein and therefore plasma level falls in patients receiving warfarin. It is activated by thrombin and in association with protein S inactivates the active forms of factor VIIIC and factor V. Plasma levels fall in DIC as a consequence of increased consumption of the protein.

53 A B C

Fungal arthritis is a rare disorder but a long delay in diagnosis is usual, frequently resulting in irreversible joint destruction. In non-endemic areas infection is predominantly seen in compromised hosts. Most cases result from direct extension from a bony focus, examples include maduromycoses, coccidioidomycosis and blastomycosis.

54 D

Proliferative diabetic retinopathy is treated initially by pan-retinal photocoagulation, not directed at the abnormal vessels. Rubeosis iridis is a feature of new vessels on the iris. All microvascular complications are exceptionally rare at presentation in IDDM. Unfortunately, pregnancy may lead to a deterioration in pre-existing retinopathy. Patients may continue to drive provided that they fulfil the requirements for visual fields and acuity.

55 B

A unilateral dorsolateral pontine lesion will produce an ipsilateral Horner's syndrome, ataxia and contralateral loss of pain and temperature sensation in the limbs. A unilateral paramedian pontine lesion will produce ipsilateral sixth and lower motor neurone seventh cranial nerve palsies and contralateral loss of touch and proprioception in the limbs. A unilateral basal pontine lesion will produce ipsilateral sixth and lower motor neurone seventh nerve palsies and contralateral hemiplegia (Millard Gubler syndrome). In addition, upper motor neurone fibres to the contralateral seventh cranial nerve nucleus may produce a contralateral upper motor neurone seventh cranial nerve palsy. A contralateral hemiplegia occurs since the pyramidal tract decussates in the medulla. The third cranial nerve nucleus lies within the midbrain. Bilateral lesions above the medulla are required to produce a pseudobulbar palsy.

56 B C D

In constrictive pericarditis the patient is characteristically breathless on exertion but not at rest; orthopnoea is slight or absent. Ascites is much more prominent than peripheral oedema. The jugular venous pulse typically rises on inspiration (Kussmauls sign) and there is a sharp and marked y descent in early diastole, coinciding with the third heart sound or pericardial knock. In long standing cases of constrictive pericarditis from any cause, calcification is common. The patient is usually in atrial fibrillation.

57 A C E

Haemolytic anaemia is a rare adverse drug effect. Dapsone causes a non-immune type of haemolytic anaemia which is more likely in patients with G6PD deficiency. Methyl dopa stimulates production of autoantibodies which give a positive Coomb's test in up to 20% of patients but haemolysis is rare. Sulphasalazine also induces haemolysis by an immune mechanism.

58 A B C D E

Migrating parasitic larvae are responsible for tissue oedema in trichinosis and gnathostomiasis. Adult loa-loa worms are occasionally seen crossing the conjunctiva and in addition cause Calabar swellings which are not infrequently periorbital. Chagas disease (American trypanosomiasis) is transmitted by the contaminated faeces of infected reduviid bugs and an inflammatory lesion often occurs at the portal of entry. This may be the conjunctiva, resulting in Romana's sign.

59 D

Over 99% of thyroxine is bound to circulating proteins, predominantly thyroxine binding globulin which is produced by the liver. Thyroglobulin is a protein in the colloid of the thyroid follicles and does not normally appear in the blood. Its measurement may be useful in thyroid carcinoma where it is used as a tumour marker. Triiodothyronine is produced largely in the periphery as a consequence of monodeiodination of thyroxine which has a half life of about 36 hours. TSH is a potent stimulus to thyroid growth in the normal individual and is responsible for the goitre of iodine deficiency and dyshormonogenesis (negative feedback).

60 C D

Clostridium difficile is present in approximately 5% of the adult population and the onset and severity of colitis is unrelated to the length of antibiotic treatment. The histological changes are diagnostic. Metronidazole is recognized as the drug of first choice but should be given orally whenever possible.

ANSWERS TO PRACTICE EXAM 4

1   A C D E
Asbestosis can cause calcified pleural plaques. Chickenpox causes fine nodular calcification. Silicosis causes 'eggshell' calcification in lymph nodes. Collections of haemosiderin containing macrophages can enlarge and calcify in the lung fields in mitral stenosis. The infiltrates in farmers' lung do not calcify.

2   A B C D E
Pregnancy (chorea gravidarum) and oral contraceptive medication may precipitate chorea. Amphetamines, tricyclic antidepressants, lithium, phenytoin, carbamazepine and cimetidine may also induce chorea. Tardive dyskinesia may follow long term neuroleptic medication. Systemic lupus erythematosus, Huntington's disease, Wilson's disease and hyperthyroidism also cause chorea.

3   A B C D
The tricyclic antidepressants have a number of important side effects. There are five main groups. Autonomic effects: dry mouth, blurred vision, urinary retention, constipation, postural hypotension, tachycardia and increased sweating. Tricyclics are contraindicated in glaucoma. Psychiatric effects: sedation, acute confusional states. Cardiovascular effects: ECG changes include prolonged PR and QT intervals, depressed ST segment and flattened T waves. Ventricular tachycardias may develop, usually where there is heart disease. Neurological effects: fine tremor, incoordination, headaches, epileptic fits, peripheral neuropathy. Other: allergic rashes, cholestatic jaundice and agranulocytosis. Tricyclic anti-depressants may be used in patients with ischaemic heart disease, with caution. They are safe in patients anticoagulated with warfarin.

4   A B

Characteristic features of hypoparathyroidism include calcification of the basal ganglia (and possible Parkinsonism), carpopedal spasm, cataract, and papilloedema. Biochemistry typically shows elevated serum phosphate with low calcium and alkaline phosphatase. Delayed tendon relaxation is a feature of hypothyroidism: muscular excitability and hyperreflexia are seen in hypocalcaemic states.

5   A D

Causes of hypokalaemia with acidosis include renal tubular acidosis, ureterocolic fistula (spontaneous or surgical) and acetazolamide treatment. Hypokalaemic alkalosis is a feature of bulimia and Conn's syndrome. Methanol poisoning typically produces features of metabolic acidosis with hyperkalaemia and low plasma bicarbonate.

6   C E

Hepatitis C is an RNA flavivirus. It is less likely to produce jaundice than hepatitis B but a greater percentage of those infected will have a chronic active hepatitis that will progress to cirrhosis, perhaps taking 20 years or more. Hepatocellular carcinoma is well recognized. Hepatitis D only complicates hepatitis B infection.

7   A B C

Weakness of triceps is unusual in a radial nerve palsy as the lesion is typically distal to the triceps branch. The radial nerve (C5,6,7,8) supplies triceps (C7), brachioradialis (C5,6), supinator (C6,7) and wrist, finger and thumb extensors (C7,8). Flexor carpi radialis (C6,7) is supplied by the median nerve (C6,7,8,T1). A C7 nerve root lesion is associated with sensory loss affecting the middle finger. A radial nerve palsy causes an absent brachioradialis reflex (C5,6), and only if the lesion is very proximal will the triceps reflex (C7) be lost.

8   A B C D E

A pedunculated left atrial myxoma may fall into the mitral orifice and obstruct blood flow into the left ventricle; thus syncope and acute pulmonary oedema may occur. Less often the findings resemble those produced by combined mitral stenosis and regurgitation or even pure mitral regurgitation. Embolic manifestations are common resulting in stroke, peripheral gangrene etc. There is often a raised sedimentation rate and high serum globulin.

9   B E

Plasmodium vivax causes benign tertian malaria. The hypnozoite stage is responsible for relapses and should be eradicated with primaquine in those who are not G6PD deficient. Chloroquine resistance is generally only seen in falciparum malaria but is now also being seen with *P. vivax* in Oceania.

10   A C E

Alzheimer's disease and Pick's disease are associated with a cortical distribution of pathology. Binswanger's disease is due to multiple small infarcts within the subcortical white matter. Normal pressure hydrocephalus, Parkinson's disease and Wilson's disease are also associated with subcortical dementia.

11   A B C E

Cheyne-Stokes respiration (periods of apnoea alternating with a series of breaths of increasing then decreasing amplitude) is usually due to brain stem compression with raised intracranial pressure. It may also occur as a result of metabolic upsets (such as cardiac, respiratory or renal failure) and as a result of CNS depressant drug poisoning. In diabetic ketoacidotic coma, the respirations are deep and sighing (Kussmaul).

12   D

Urobilinogen is present in the urine of normal subjects. An excess of urobilinogen can be detected by Ehrlich's aldehyde reagent. Distinction from porphobilinogen is by solubility in aqueous and non-aqueous phases. An increase of urobilinogen in the urine occurs in hepato-cellular dysfunction; urobilinogen disappears from the urine in intrahepatic obstruction. Urobilinogenuria is also found with the increased bilirubin formation of haemolysis. Mild haemolysis is a feature of pernicious anaemia.

13   A

The carcinoid syndrome, due to tumour overproduction of serotonin (5-HT) may be treated with specific 5-HT antagonists or octreotide (somatostatin analogue). Right sided heart lesions are characteristic (tricuspid and pulmonary valve thickening) and more likely with bronchial lesions. Flushing, wheeze and diarrhoea are the usual complaints, pallor and sweating being better associated with phaeochromocytoma. There may be long term survival (>10 years). Diagnosis is best made by 24 hour urine collections for 5HIAA, a metabolite of 5-HT.

14   A D E

Minoxidil is a prodrug, the active metabolite of which dilates arterioles selectively rather than veins. Inactivation is by further liver metabolism. A compensatory increase in heart rate prompts combination therapy. Oedema is common and most patients require a diuretic. Hypertrichosis is troublesome in women: it resolves about 3 months after drug withdrawal. The tachycardia can induce angina but the ECG changes are seldom accompanied by symptoms.

15   A B C

ARF may follow ACE inhibitor treatment in patients with pre-existent renovascular disease or renal hypoperfusion; renal size is normal or kidneys may be swollen in ARF. Haemolytic anaemia occurs in haemolytic-uraemic syndrome and certain vasculitides (e.g. SLE). Reflux uropathy accounts for 30% of cases of CRF, but a history of urinary infection is only documented in 25% of cases. An aortic aneurysm may involve the renal arteries, resulting in either CRF or ARF if acute thrombosis of the vessels occurs or the aneurysm ruptures.

16   A B

Methotrexate is an antimetabolite which inhibits the conversion of folic acid to dihydrofolic acid and of this to tetrahydrofolic acid (essential to DNA synthesis). Alkylating agents denature preformed DNA: they include mustine, chlorambucil, melphalan and cyclophosphamide. Vinblastine and vincristine are vinca alkaloids which disrupt microtubular proteins and interfere with metaphase in dividing cells. Cytosine arabinoside is a pyrimidine analogue and azathioprine is a purine analogue: both inhibit DNA synthesis. Anti-cancer drugs have greatest activity and toxicity in rapidly dividing tissues where there is less time for DNA repair or synthesis between cell divisions.

17   A B D

Transforming growth factor beta is a 25 kD homodimeric peptide that can occur in at least three isoforms, each with discrete biological effects. It is released from platelets during degranulation and is able to induce its own production from monocytes. It is intimately involved in the inflammatory response promoting wound healing and modulating the immune response by suppressing lymphocyte proliferation.

18   A E

In HOCM the onset of atrial fibrillation commonly precipitates congestive cardiac failure which is poorly tolerated. The late systolic murmur is maximal at the left sternal edge. Trinitrin increases outflow obstruction. Propranolol therapy results in symptomatic improvement in many patients but it does not prevent the complication of sudden death. Echocardiography detects septal wall hypertrophy and abnormal systolic anterior motion of the anterior leaflet of the mitral valve.

19 A B D E
The side effects of digoxin are protean and often affect elderly patients who have reduced tolerance to the drug. Gastrointestinal symptoms are prominent with anorexia, vomiting, abdominal pain, diarrhoea and weight loss. Confusion, delirium and seizures may occur. Visual symptoms include alterations in colour vision and even blindness. A wide variety of ventricular and supraventricular rhythms may occur and can be difficult to treat.

20 A B
Depression and delusional symptoms occur in Cushing's syndrome, whatever the aetiology. Hypertension is a consequence of ACTH stimulation of cortisol secretion which has some mineralocorticoid action. Hirsutism (androgen dependent hair) but not hypertrichosis (generalised hairiness) may complicate excess androgen secretion from pituitary dependent disease or adrenal tumour. Glucocorticoid excess in children typically slows growth. Polycythaemia is a rare accompaniment but anaemia is not a recognized manifestation.

21 A B C D E
A clinical picture resembling infectious mononucleosis, including the presence of atypical lymphocytes in the peripheral blood, can be seen at the time of primary HIV infection. ITP has been reported with increasing frequency in HIV-infected persons. Cytopenia of all peripheral blood cell lineages can be seen in HIV infection. Morphological features of myelodysplasia such as megaloblastic erythropoiesis are commonly identified in the bone marrow smears obtained from HIV-positive individuals. Circulating immunoglobulins with antiphospholipid activity such as the lupus anticoagulant have been demonstrated in patients with HIV infection, particularly in association with acute infection such as with *Pneumocystis carinii*.

22 C E
Chickenpox encephalitis is an immune phenomenon occurring with the resolution of skin lesions. The clinical features are cerebellar and the process is self limiting. Herpes simplex encephalitis predominantly

affects the temporal lobes and in 90% of cases is due to HSV 1. Encephalitis as well as transverse myelitis and Guillain Barre syndrome may complicate mycoplasma infection.

23 A B C D

Lesch-Nyhan syndrome is an X-linked disorder in which there is deficiency of hypoxanthine guanosine phosphoribosyl transferase. There is overproduction of urate, gout, neurological disease and self mutilation. The serum uric acid is elevated in myeloproliferative disorders such as polycythaemia rubra vera. Hyperuricaemia is also associated with hyperparathyroidism and hypothyroidism but not with thyrotoxicosis. Hydroxybutyrate accumulation in fasting inhibits renal tubular urate secretion.

24 B C D

A unilateral paramedian midbrain lesion will produce an ipsilateral third cranial nerve palsy and contralateral ataxia (Benedikt's syndrome) due to involvement of the red nucleus which interrupts the dentato-rubro-thalamic tract. A unilateral basal midbrain lesion will produce an ipsilateral third cranial nerve palsy and contralateral hemiplegia (Weber's syndrome). A unilateral dorsolateral midbrain lesion will produce an ipsilateral Horner's syndrome, contralateral total sensory loss and ipsilateral ataxia due to involvement of the superior cerebellar peduncle. The sixth cranial nerve nucleus is located in the pons. Bilateral lesions are required to produce a pseudobulbar palsy.

25 B C D

Crackles are heard in bronchiectasis, pulmonary oedema, left ventricular failure and pulmonary fibrosis as in extrinsic allergic alveolitis and sarcoidosis.

26 A B

Diazepam and the other benzodiazepines have many of the qualitative features of the barbiturates. The difference is in their margin of safety. Tolerance and dependence occur with prolonged use. The ratio between anxiolytic and respiratory depressant dose for the barbiturates is small and that for diazepam is large. When the use of diazepam is restricted to short periods the risk of barbiturate-like hazards is virtually nil. Diazepam does not interact with warfarin. Diazepam binds to the benzodiazepine receptor and enhances GABA facilitated inhibitory synaptic transmission. Diazepam itself has a short plasma half life (8 hours) but its main metabolites (nordiazepam, oxazepam) are active and long acting.

27 A D E

A D E may all result in a dry tap due to increased reticulin. Aplasia may be patchy and Reed-Sternberg cells are difficult to identify in a hypercellular aspirate. Histology makes interpretation of morphology of the erythroid series difficult.

28 C D

BIH usually occurs in overweight young females and is associated with pregnancy, oral contraceptives, tetracyclines and nalidixic acid. Hypervitaminosis A is a rare cause. BIH may cause a sixth cranial nerve palsy (false localising sign of raised intracranial pressure) and any of the signs associated with papilloedema. The lateral ventricles are usually normal or 'slit-like'.

29 A D E

This indicates that the subject is capable of six times the exertion that would have been possible without it. Trained athletes are able to increase the oxygen consumption of their muscles to a greater degree than untrained individuals. Consequently, they are capable of greater exertion without increasing lactic acid production and hence contract smaller oxygen debts for a given amount of exertion. The production of lactic acid, which is inevitable with the anaerobic pathway in action, results in a lowering of the pH due to an accumulation of acid. Thus the use of the anaerobic pathway is self-limiting.

30 B E

Endothelium derived relaxation factor is nitric oxide. It is formed by endothelial cells from L-arginine and is released immediately into the microenvironment where it acts directly on guanylate cyclase to increase cyclic GMP leading to vasodilation.

31 A B C

Gastrin production is stimulated by a rise in gastric intraluminal pH (i.e. reduced acidity) such as that produced by omeprazole. Elevated gastrin levels also occur in chronic renal failure as gastrin is excreted in the urine. The elevated levels found after massive small bowel resection are unexplained. Patients with duodenal ulcers do not show significant elevations of plasma gastrin as secretion is inhibited by duodenal acidification. Very high plasma gastrin is a feature of the Zollinger-Ellison syndrome which forms part of the syndrome MEA type I.

32 A B E

The most prominent signs in the initial leptospiraemic phase of the illness are conjunctival suffusion, neck stiffness, cutaneous haemorrhages and fever. Splenomegaly may occur but is uncommon. Jaundice is common but there is only mild hepatitis. The organism can be grown in blood cultures although the diagnosis is usually made by rising serological titres.

33 B D E

The PO_2 may fall on exercise but not at rest. Lung function studies indicate a restrictive defect with reduced FVC but normal FEV1/FVC ratio, and a reduced diffusing capacity.

34 A B C D E

TGA is an ill understood disorder in which there is an abrupt onset of anterograde amnesia with repetitive questioning. It is associated with precipitating factors such as vigorous exercise, sexual intercourse, sudden temperature change and may follow vertebral angiography. It tends to last only a few hours. It is due to transient bilateral medial temporal lobe dysfunction and may have an underlying vasospastic basis. Repetitive episodes of memory disturbance with associated reduction of conscious level in an individual less than 40 years old are more suggestive of complex partial seizures of temporal lobe onset. Repetitive episodes of memory disturbance with vertigo, unsteadiness and visual disturbance are more suggestive of transient ischaemic episodes in the vertebrobasilar territory. Loss of memory and personal identity usually has an underlying psychiatric basis.

35 B C E

Guanine nucleotide binding proteins are ubiquitous proteins located at the inner aspect of cell membranes. They include a large family of proteins, including Ras oncogene. During activation, guanosine triphosphate is bound to the subunit which promotes signal transduction. Deactivation occurs through hydrolysis of GTP to GDP.

36 C

A is false, the difference in the efficacies of the two treatments (improvement rates of 77% for the active drug and 57% for the placebo) is reasonably impressive numerically. However, a formal statistical test is needed to estimate the probability of the difference occurring by chance under the null hypothesis that the two treatments are equipotent (this probability is actually approximately 1%, so the difference is statistically significant). B is false, the appropriate test of significance for comparing frequencies/

proportions is the chi-squared test; Pearson's coefficient is a measure of correlation. D is false, Student's t-test is used for continuous data. E is false, sequential analysis requires the patients to be paired and for a direct comparison of each pair to be made as the study progresses.

37 A C D

Tactful enquiry about suicidal intent may decrease the risk of suicide. The following factors are associated with an increased risk of suicide: male sex, old age, alcohol abuse, drug dependence, epilepsy, chronic physical illness (especially chronically painful conditions), bereavement, social isolation, psychiatric disorder (apart from obsessional illness), family history of suicide or depression, previous suicide attempts, unemployment.

38 B D E

The mitotic cell cycle is made up of: (a) Interphase; subdivided into G1 (the synthesis of RNA and proteins), S (replication of DNA) and G2 (synthesis of organelles); (b) Mitotic nuclear division; subdivided into protophase (chromosomes become visible and spindles are formed), metaphase (chromosomes line up at the spindle equator), anaphase (chromatids and centromeres separate) and telophase (where two new nuclear membranes are formed); (c) Cytoplasmic cleavage.

39 B

Mucosal ulcers occur in approximately 30% of patients with secondary syphilis. Tertiary disease develops three or more years after the primary stage and the skin, mucous membranes and bones are typically involved. Procaine penicillin is the treatment of choice for all stages. After treatment of primary and secondary disease the VDRL usually becomes negative whereas the TPHA remains positive.

40 B

The superior gluteal nerve (L4,5,S1) supplies gluteus minimus, medius and tensor fasciae latae. The femoral nerve (L2,3,4) supplies quadriceps femoris (rectus femoris, vastus lateralis, intermedius and medialis) and skin over the anterior and medial thigh and medial lower leg. The lateral cutaneous nerve of thigh supplies skin over the lateral aspect of thigh. Gastrocnemius is supplied by the tibial nerve, a branch of the sciatic nerve. The sciatic nerve (L4,5,S1,2,3) supplies the hamstring muscle group directly.

41 A B D

Urticaria may be a feature in many of the diseases caused by nematode or flatworm infestation (e.g. strongyloidiasis, filiariasis and schistosomiasis). The opiate drugs are histamine-releasers and salicylates can aggravate urticaria and asthma. SLE may present with urticarial vasculitis.

42 A B C D E

Co-trimoxazole is the therapy of choice and is usually given in high doses intravenously. Pentamidine is an alternative. Both are associated with a high incidence of side effects in AIDS patients. Bronchoalveolar lavage is diagnostic in 90% of cases.

43 A E

Myasthenia gravis causes fatiguable weakness of ocular, facial, bulbar and proximal limb musculature. Dysarthria and dysphagia are due to bulbar involvement whereas dysphasia is indicative of a cerebral cortical lesion. Tendon reflexes are typically preserved.

44 C

Bicuspid aortic valves have a tendency to calcify; the most common cause of aortic stenosis in the 40–60 age group (with senile calcification of a tricuspid valve becoming more common in the elderly). Although coarctation of the aorta is associated with a bicuspid aortic valve, Turner's syndrome is associated with coarctation of the aorta without bicuspid aortic valve.

45 B C E

Alport's syndrome is an hereditary glomerulonephritis (X-linked or dominant) which classically is associated with sensorineural deafness and characteristic eye lesions. It is due to mutations of the 5 chain of type IV collagen of basement membrane, which is the antigen recognized in Goodpasture's syndrome. Therefore, antiglomerular basement membrane disease can occur post renal transplant but Alport's syndrome cannot recur. The disease is rarely associated with leiomyomatosis, macrothrombocytopenia or hyperprolinaemia.

46 E

Peak bone mass is achieved in the early twenties in women and declines from there, although the rate of bone loss accelerates when the patient becomes oestrogen deficient. Flushes and sweating are due to vasomotor instability which is a consequence of oestrogen deficiency. The fall in serum oestrogen leads to a rise in circulating gonadotrophins, predominantly FSH. Bowel disturbance is not a characteristic feature of the menopause. The incidence of myocardial infarction rises slowly in the years after menopause when the protective influence of oestrogen is lost.

47 A C D E
The irritable bowel syndrome is well recognised following salmonella gastroenteritis. Although previously thought to represent abnormal neuromuscular coordination of the colon, no characteristic abnormality of large bowel motility has yet been defined. An increased awareness of colonic action is characteristic of the syndrome and may be secondary to a lowered threshold of activity in colonic afferent neurons. Dysuria, headache, low back pain and non-ulcer dyspepsia are all associated and may represent a similar underlying pathophysiology of other organs.

48 A E
Haemophilia A is inherited in an X-linked fashion but up to 30% of patients have no family history and presumably it results from spontaneous mutations. Classically the bleeding tendency results in spontaneous haemorrhage into joints and muscles, Bleeding into the skin is a feature but is less common. The deficiency of the coagulation factor VIIIC results in a defect in the intrinsic pathway of the clotting cascade, the extrinsic pathway is not affected. This produces a prolongation of the activated partial thromboplastin time (APTT) but not the prothrombin time (PT). The bleeding time is abnormal in disorders where there is a bleeding tendency due to thrombocytopenia, abnormal platelet function or vascular defects, it is unaffected by abnormalities of the coagulation cascade.

49 A B E
Indications include any evidence of bone destruction, renal disease, renal stone formation and very high uric acid levels. It would not be usual to initiate hypouricaemic therapy until three or more acute attacks had occurred.

50 B E
Microalbuminuria, defined as detectable albuminuria (30–300 mcg/min or roughly 25-250 mg/24 hr) below the clearly proteinuric range is best assessed with a timed overnight specimen as 24 hour specimens may be affected by orthostatic proteinuria. Angiotensin converting enzyme inhibitors reduce protein excretion and delay development of renal impairment even in normotensive individuals. Microalbuminuria should raise the level of suspicion for proliferative retinopathy but this is not universal. In NIDDM patients there is a strong association between the finding of microalbuminuria and development of macrovascular disease.

51 None correct

The onset of Parkinson's disease is usually between the ages of 55 and 70. Tremor is most pronounced at rest and rigidity is equally pronounced in limb flexion and extension. Broad based gait disturbance and early urinary incontinence are features of normal pressure hydrocephalus.

52 B C

In left ventricular failure, interstitial pulmonary oedema interferes with gas transfer. Alveolar PCO_2 is increased only when the fluid has entered terminal airways. As the left ventricle fails, left ventricular end-diastolic pressure and pulmonary venous pressure rise. X-ray changes may antedate auscultatory findings by 24 hours, depending on the rapidity of onset.

53 B D E

Drug conjugates are water soluble and allow elimination by the kidneys. Some drugs such as warfarin form hydroxylated metabolites which are sufficiently water soluble for excretion without the need for conjugation. Isoniazid is acetylated. Temazepam forms a glucuronide. Paracetamol forms glucuronide and sulphate conjugates. Phenytoin is hydroxylated then conjugated with glucuronides.

54 B D E

Amantadine is active against influenza A and administered *prophylactically* is as effective as vaccination. The role of AZT in asymptomatic HIV infection is still controversial but no trial has shown proven benefit for patients with a CD4 count of over 500.

55 A B E

Unilateral exophthalmos should raise the suspicion of an orbital tumour and is invariably an indication for CT scanning of the orbit, even in the presence of Graves' disease (where eye signs may be asymmetrical or unilateral). Wegener's more typically causes destruction of bone in the midline but may rarely lead to exophthalmos. Cigarette smoking exacerbates Graves' ophthalmopathy but does not itself cause exophthalmos. Exophthalmos means protrusion of the orbital contents and though there may be enophthalmos in Horner's syndrome, this does not imply contralateral exophthalmos.

56 A B

In both Crohn's disease and radiation enteritis affecting the terminal ileum, a failure of bile salt resorption may occur resulting in an overall decrease in the circulating bile acid pool. Eventually, inadequate production of bile acids leads to malabsorption of fat. Fat malabsorption in cystic fibrosis occurs as a result of impaired digestion. Mucosal lesions of the upper small intestine, such as coeliac disease and giardiasis, lead directly to malabsorption of fat without evidence of bile acid deficiency.

57 A B D E
Cryoglobulins are immunoglobulin molecules that reversibly precipitate at low temperature. They are found in patients with myeloma and associated disorders but are also seen in infections, connective tissue diseases, lymphoproliferative diseases and miscellaneous disorders. Monoclonal proteins are usually associated with myeloma. Mixed cryoglobulins are most frequently found consisting of IgM and IgG. The symptoms are usually fairly mild and include cold induced urticaria, Raynaud's and cutaneous ulcers. Polyarthralgia independent purpura may also be present. Circulating immune complexes and occlusion of vessels are important in the pathogenesis of the disease.

58 A B
The haemopoietic growth factors are glycoprotein hormones that regulate the proliferation and differentiation of haemopoietic progenitor cells and the function of mature cells. They include erythropoietin, granulocyte macrophage colony stimulating factor (GM-CSF), granulocyte colony stimulating factor (G-CSF), macrophage colony stimulating factor (M-CSF) and interleukin 3. Each growth factor is encoded by a single gene on a number of different chromosomes. These factors are unrelated to the immunoglobulin superfamily.

59 A
Accelerated hypertension due to renal artery stenosis is caused by hyper-reninaemia and consequent hyperaldosteronism, the latter resulting in hypokalaemic alkalosis. Until significant hypertensive damage occurs in the contralateral kidney, renal function, both tubular and glomerular, is maintained even when the blood pressure is lowered by the angiotensin convertase inhibitor, captopril. Increased pyelographic concentration may occur in the affected kidney.

60 A D E
In the absence of coarse brain disease the presence of Schneider's first rank symptoms point to a diagnosis of schizophrenia. They are:
(1) Specific types of auditory hallucination (audible thoughts, voices talking about the patient in the third person, voices commenting on actions (running commentary)).

(2) Passivity phenomena (breakdown of ego-boundaries), thought insertion, withdrawal and broadcast, made acts and feelings (somatic passivity). (3) Delusions (primary delusions or delusional perceptions).

ANSWERS TO PRACTICE EXAM 5

1 A

The common peroneal nerve and tibial nerve are branches of the sciatic nerve. A common peroneal nerve palsy causes weakness of foot eversion and dorsiflexion (foot-drop). Foot inversion is not completely lost as tibialis posterior is supplied by the tibial nerve. Skin over the medial aspect of the lower leg is supplied by the saphenous branch of the femoral nerve and that over the lateral aspect of lower leg by the superficial branch of the common peroneal nerve. A sciatic nerve lesion causes loss of the ankle reflex.

2 D E

The bullous pemphigoid antigen is part of the hemidesmosome which links the epidermis to the dermis: the desmosome links keratinocytes together. Keratinocytes, melanocytes and Langerhans cells are found in the epidermis; melanin with melanosomes is passed from melanocytes into keratinocytes. Eccrine sweat glands are most profuse on the forehead, palms, soles and axillae and are innervated by cholinergic sympathetic fibres.

3 A B C E

Pulmonary eosinophilia may occur with a number of drugs, including nitrofurantoin, Salazopyrin, sulphonylureas and PAS. Loffler's syndrome is a transient pulmonary infiltration which usually resolves within weeks and may be produced by drugs or intestinal parasites.

4 A D

Limb weakness affects proximal limb musculature whereas pseudo-hypertrophy affects more distal musculature of the calves and forearms. Limb contractures may be a late clinical manifestation of Duchenne muscular dystrophy but are an early feature of Emery-Dreifuss muscular dystrophy (X-linked recessive). EMGs show a typically myopathic appearance.

5 B C D

The first heart sound is characteristically soft; when loud it excludes severe mitral regurgitation. The third heart sound and diastolic murmur (in the absence of any stenosis) reflect rapid diastolic filling of the left ventricle. Left atrial distension in systole may produce a left sternal heave. The second heart sound is usually normal; with severe regurgitation early aortic valve closure causes wide (but not reversed) splitting of the second sound. A mid systolic click suggests mitral leaflet prolapse as the cause of the regurgitation. Acute mitral regurgitation, which may produce an apical thrill, may be due to papillary muscle infarction and rupture.

6   B E

In MS, breakdown of the blood brain barrier precedes both symptoms and MRI signs of demyelination. Perivascular helper T cells are found in acute MS lesions and there is abnormal MHC class II expression on macrophages and astrocytes resulting in antigen presentation. The resulting T cell proliferation and activation of B cells with macrophages leads to demyelination by killing of oligodendrocytes which have little, if any, proliferative capacity. The loss of myelin prevents saltatory conduction between the nodes of Ranvier.

7   C D

In Turner's syndrome, there is loss of all or part of one of the X chromosomes and in rare cases there may be translocation of the genetic material to an autosome, hence other karyotypes are possible. Turner girls are short prepubertally due to an associated skeletal dysplasia and fail to undergo the normal pubertal growth spurt due to oestrogen deficiency. This leads to poor breast development and a small uterus. Both organs enlarge when appropriate sex steroid replacement treatment is given. Serum FSH is high as a result of negative feedback.

8   B E

Patients with the syndrome of inappropriate ADH secretion are euvolaemic and do not develop ascites. Ascites and oedema are recognized features of kwashiorkor rather than marasmus. Hepatocellular carcinoma and peritoneal mesothelioma may both produce ascites. Restrictive cardiomyopathy and constrictive pericarditis are rare causes of ascites.

9   A D

Thrombocytopenia occurs in approximately 5% of patients receiving heparin in therapeutic doses. Paradoxically arterial and venous thrombosis occurs in up to 20% of patients with heparin-induced thrombocytopenia and is associated with a 50% mortality rate. Osteoporosis and alopecia are recognized adverse effects of long-term administration with heparin.

Heparin can be used with relative safety in pregnancy, coumarin anticoagulants are suspected to be teratogenic when used in the first trimester.

10 A

Hypermobility generally arises because of laxity in periarticular tissues rather than bony or joint damage. Acromegaly is associated with an increase in joint space due to cartilage overgrowth but this does not lead to hypermobility.

11 A

Maculopathy is certainly more common in the older patient with NIDDM but may occur in young patients as well. The patient may be registered blind because of the damage to the very sensitive macular area. However, even though the patient may be unable to read, they may retain excellent peripheral (navigational) vision. Treatment of maculopathy is usually with small, focal laser burns to the macular area, avoiding the fovea, in contrast to treatment for proliferative retinopathy which usually involves several thousand burns to the peripheral retina. Drusen are a normal feature in some patients. Hard exudates, often in rings (circinates) are characteristic of diabetic maculopathy. Painful visual loss is not a feature of maculopathy and suggests glaucoma, uveitis or corneal ulcer.

12 C D

Dysphasia is due to a lesion in the dominant cerebral cortex. Hemianopia indicates a lesion of the optic tract, radiation or occipital cortex. Dysarthria is most likely to be due to subcortical, midbrain or brain stem pathology. Upper motor neurone signs may be produced by cerebral, midbrain, brain stem or cord pathology.

13 A B D

Pericarditis is a late finding in patients with severe renal impairment. In hypothyroidism, other cardiological abnormalities include low ECG voltage, bradycardia and ischaemic heart disease. Carditis, including pericarditis is one of the major diagnostic criteria of acute rheumatic fever. Subarachnoid haemorrhage may cause widespread ST segment changes in the ECG but this is not due to pericarditis.

14 A B D

Reduced cardiac output and antagonism of circulating adrenaline at vascular beta-adrenoceptors sub serving vasodilation combine to reduce peripheral blood flow. Not only does restoration of normal blood glucose take longer but also the symptoms of hypoglycaemia are partially masked. Physiological tremor is enhanced by agonists at beta-adrenoceptors. Vivid dreams are common: hallucinations and confusional states also occur. Propranolol has been used to reduce bleeding from oesophageal varices.

15 B

A neutrophil leucocytosis is in general suggestive of bacterial, rickettsial and spirochaetal infections. In dengue (flavavirus), brucellosis and typhoid fever the neutrophil count is usually normal or low.

16 A B C E

Menorrhagia and normochromic anaemia are not uncommon complications of hypothyroidism. Remember that menorrhagia may lead to a microcytic picture and associated vitamin B12 deficiency may cause a macrocytic blood film. Clinically significant ascites and cerebellar ataxia are rare. Clubbing (thyroid acropachy) and pretibial myxoedema are rare manifestations of autoimmune thyrotoxicosis (Graves' disease) and usually occur in association with severe exophthalmic eye disease.

17 B

H. pylori is a Gram-negative organism that survives in the mucous layer of the gastric mucosa. It most often produces non-erosive antral gastritis and can be found in 90% of duodenal ulcer sufferers. The urease breath test is used to confirm the presence of the organism.

18 A C E

Hypocomplementaemia results from immune complex formation and complement consumption in SLE, cryoglobulinaemia and post infective glomerulonephritis. Hypocomplementaemia can also result from non-immune complement activation as in severe sepsis, pancreatitis and athero-embolism. Pregnancy and chronic inflammatory states lead to an increase in serum complement levels.

19 B D E

Apoptosis is programmed cell death and leads to the removal of 'unwanted cells' (and their potentially injurious contents) without tissue necrosis or injury. It is involved in a wide variety of important biological processes; including embryological remodelling, thymic selection of lymphocytes and tumour involution. The biochemical 'hallmark' is internucleosomal chromatin cleavage, resulting in condensation of nuclear chromatin as a result of endogenous endonuclease activation.

20 A D E

The ureter and bladder are lined with transitional epithelium whereas the vas deferens is lined with columnar epithelium. The sympathetic nerve supply to the ureter is from spinal cord segments L1 and L2. Remember that there is no sympathetic outflow below L2.

21 E

Puerperal psychosis usually begins within the first one to two weeks, but rarely in the first two days. There are three main types of clinical picture: acute organic, affective (depressive or manic) and schizophrenic. The most common presentation is depressive. The onset is usually acute and the prognosis good. The risk of recurrence in subsequent pregnancies is between 1:3 and 1:7.

22 A B C

Lymphomas, retrosternal thyroid, terato-dermoids pericardial cysts and aneurysms of the ascending aorta all typically occur in the anterior mediastinum. Neurogenic tumours, paravertebral abscesses and descending aneurysms are posterior.

23 B D

Essential tremor is most pronounced with outstretched arms (sustained posture) and is typically relieved by alcohol. A Parkinson's disease tremor is most pronounced at rest and a cerebellar tremor with movement (intention). Anxiety may exacerbate both an essential and Parkinson's disease tremor.

24 C E

Negligible evidence supports the numerous claims of differences in the pharmacodynamics of the dozen or so available benzodiazepines. They do however differ in their duration of action. Triazolam, temazepam and oxazepam are short-acting (plasma concentration half time less than 10 hours). The remainder persist in the body for a long time (e.g. diazepam and its active metabolites) with a half time of up to 3 days in the elderly. Metabolism is mainly by oxidation then to glucuronide conjugates. The increase in body sway predisposes to falls, especially in the elderly.

25 C

In sarcoidosis with hypercalcaemia, PTH levels are suppressed by the hypercalcaemia, which is in turn due to excess vitamin D activity as a consequence of increased 25 hydroxylation of cholecalciferol in granulomatous tissue. In primary hyperparathyroidism, the PTH level is usually high but may be in the normal range but inappropriately so in the presence of hypercalcaemia (which should suppress it). PTH stimulates renal 1-alpha hydroxylase and in the human consists of 84 amino acids. Many peptide hormones are now measured by two-site immunoradiometric or non-isotopic methods rather than the older and less sensitive displacement radioimmunoassay.

26 A C
Carbon dioxide retention in chronic respiratory disease leads to renal conservation of bicarbonate to maintain plasma pH. Carpopedal spasm may be a feature of hypocalcaemia and both metabolic and respiratory alkalosis. 21 hydroxylase deficiency leads to a mild metabolic acidosis in the untreated state (low plasma bicarbonate) and this will also be observed in primary hyperparathyroidism and ureterosigmoidostomy.

27 A B C
Encephalopathy following therapeutic paracentesis is usually reversible and is uncommon. Its development is unrelated to the type of plasma volume expander chosen. Intravenous saline precipitates fluid retention and ascites in patients with cirrhosis.

28 C E
The gag reflex is usually present or pathologically brisk. Wasting of the tongue indicates lower motor neurone involvement and together with the upper motor neurone signs of pseudobulbar palsy suggests motor neurone disease (progressive bulbar palsy). Syringobulbia causes a 'true' bulbar palsy due to involvement of the IXth, Xth and XIIth cranial nerve nuclei from below. Pseudobulbar palsy is due to bilateral lesions above the IXth, Xth and XIIth cranial nuclei and may be due to cerebrovascular disease, multiple sclerosis or motor neurone disease.

29 A E
Infective endocarditis may result in an immune-complex nephritis. Combined benzylpenicillin and gentamicin is the treatment of choice in *Streptococcus faecalis* endocarditis. Invasive procedures such as sigmoidoscopy and cytoscopy result in bacteraemia and increase the risk of endocarditis in susceptible subjects. Atrial septal defect does not predispose to infective endocarditis. Echocardiography cannot be used to rule out endocarditis.

30 A B C E
Hepatitis C causes chronic hepatitis in at least 50% of those infected.

Transmission is primarily via blood products and needle sharing. Second generation ELISA kits for hepatitis C antibodies now give reliable results. Positive results are a marker of prior exposure only and liver biopsy or PCR for hepatitis C RNA are required to establish the presence of active disease.

31 None correct
Alzheimer's disease is the most common cause of dementia and the majority (90%) of cases occur sporadically. Amnesia and spatial dysfunction are typical early clinical features and social graces are usually maintained until late in the disease. The underlying pathology predominantly affects the temporal and parietal cortices. Extrapyramidal rigidity, long tract signs and myoclonus are all late clinical manifestations. The EEG is typically abnormal.

32 A B D
Lung compliance is a static measure of lung and chest recoil and is expressed as a change in lung volume per unit change in airway pressure. Since it is a static measure, it cannot be determined by using a peak flow meter. It is approximately half of normal in a person with one lung, as the lung volume is approximately half.

33 B D E
Reticulocyte response to bleeding or iron therapy is rarely higher than 5%. Spherocytosis produces crises following infection/stress. Sideroblastosis produces ineffective erythropoiesis with a low reticulocyte count. The anaemia of lead poisoning is not due to haemolysis but impaired haem-synthesis; however red cell survival is decreased and acute haemolytic anaemia occasionally occurs. Methyldopa produces a 20% incidence of positive Coomb's test but haemolytic anaemia is rare.

34 A B
Despite the fact that it is an autosomal dominant condition, more women than men are affected in AIP, probably as a result of the effect of oestrogens. Increased urinary porphobilinogen is characteristic as a result of reduced activity of the enzyme porphobilinogen deaminase. Photosensitive metabolites are not produced in this condition. Characteristic clinical features include peripheral neuropathy, tachycardia, hypertension, abdominal pain. Mononeuropathies are not characteristic although a radial nerve palsy may be seen in the related condition of lead poisoning (some similar clinical and biochemical features). Acute attacks of AIP may be characterized by hyponatraemia due to inappropriate ADH secretion.

35 B C D E

Less than 20% is absorbed after oral dosage. Enema administration is effective. Prostaglandin synthesis in vitro is suppressed not only by the salicylate metabolite but also by the parent compound. Recognized adverse effects include agranulocytosis and reversible oligospermia.

36 E

Digoxin undergoes renal elimination and toxic concentrations develop if given in normal doses in patients with chronic renal failure. The other agents largely undergo hepatic excretion and standard doses can be used safely in renal impairment.

37 C D

Endothelial-leucocyte adhesion molecules control leucocyte transmigration to sites of inflammation. They include selectin-carbohydrate interactions, immunoglobulin super family member cell adhesion molecules (IgCAMs) that bind to integrins and CD31 that is capable of homophilic interaction between endothelial and leucocyte CD31.

38 A B C D E

The right coronary artery is found in a groove between the right atrium and right ventricle. It gives off a branch to the A-V node and goes on to supply the inferior aspect of the left ventricle via the posterior descending artery in the majority of patients. It also supplies the right ventricle.

39 A C

Enterohepatic recirculation is the process whereby some drugs are excreted in the bile and then reabsorbed from the gastrointestinal tract back into the circulation. If drugs are excreted as conjugates the conjugate must be broken down by bacterial enzymes to release the parent drug.

40 A B C E

Metyrapone inhibits the enzyme 11 beta hydroxylase, the final step in cortisol synthesis. Finasteride is a competitive inhibitor of 5 alpha reductase, which converts testosterone to the active dihydrotestosterone. This agent is effective in benign and malignant prostatic disease. Enalaprilat is the active form of enalapril, which inhibits the angiotensin converting enzyme. Pyridostigmine is a competitive inhibitor of the enzyme cholinesterase and is used in the management of myasthenia gravis. Pralidoxime is used to reactivate cholinesterase following organophosphorous poisoning (sheep dip, insecticide).

41 D

Phaeochromocytoma is the ten percent tumour (10% bilateral, 10% malignant and 10% extra-adrenal). Constipation is common, as are the more usual hypertension, sweating and tachycardia. Tumour localisation with modern CT scanning is usually adequate although 131-Iodine labelled MIBG may be required for extra-adrenal tumours. Associated medullary thyroid carcinoma may be a feature of MEN type 2 syndrome. Alpha blockade is the most important initial treatment and only when this has been achieved is it safe to undertake beta blockade.

42 B C D E

The predominant haemoglobin is type F in all neonates: the thalassaemic state appears later as the child converts from Hb.F to Hb.A. Widespread marrow hyperplasia results in bony overgrowth. The prognosis is grave and many children fail to survive into adult life.

43 A

Although lymphopenia, and in particular CD4 lymphocyte depletion, in HIV patients is associated with oropharyngeal and oesophageal candidiasis, candidaemia and deep infection is principally a problem in neutropenic patients. Endocarditis is usually left sided and should be considered in cases of culture-negative endocarditis.

44 C E

Severe poisoning, when lithium is taken in overdose, is characterized by diarrhoea, coma, seizures, muscle tremor, cerebellar ataxia and nephrogenic diabetes insipidus. There may also be apparent hyperkalaemia.

45 B C E

Ankylosing spondylitis is associated with fibro-bullous disease of the apices. Pleurisy with or without effusion can complicate any collagen vascular disorder. Basal pneumonia in systemic sclerosis results from oesophageal dysfunction and aspiration. Yellow nails demonstrate a deficiency of lymphatics and the effusion is not chylous. The most frequent primaries to cause lymphangitis are stomach, pancreas, breast and prostate.

46 A B

Ipsilateral twelfth cranial nerve palsy, contralateral hemiplegia and contralateral loss of touch and joint position sense are typical of a medial medullary lesion. Ipsilateral Horner's syndrome and ataxia are features of a lateral medullary lesion.

47 A B C E

Hypokalaemia (occasionally occurring with prolonged use of thiazide diuretics) causes a prominent U wave, T wave flattening, and later ST depression and T wave inversion. Acute pericarditis causes concave upward ST elevation and chronic pericarditis may reduce voltages. The strain pattern of left ventricular hypertrophy shows ST depression and digoxin toxicity shows ST depression with the reversed tick appearance. Syndrome X is characterized by anginal-type chest pain, angiographically-normal coronary arteries and ST depression on exercise.

48 C D E

Hydralazine lowers blood pressure and slow acetylators have a more marked response. Isoniazid hepatitis may be related to a metabolite since it is more common in fast acetylators. The remaining adverse effects are dose dependent and are more commonly seen in slow acetylators.

49 A D

Falciparum malaria is the most virulent of the four types of malaria and splenomegaly is an important clinical sign. Acute renal failure is common. There is no dormant liver stage as in vivax, ovale or malariae and recurrence of fever after one year is rare. Tertian periodicity does occur but is far from characteristic.

50 A B C D E

Hypercalcaemia may occur in patients with extensive Paget's disease when immobilised or when osteosarcoma develops. Deafness may be due to either direct Pagetic involvement of the ossicles of the inner ear or to pressure on the eighth cranial nerve by Pagetic bone. Overgrowth of Pagetic bone at the base of the skull may lead to brain stem compression. Angioid streaks in the retina are found very rarely in Paget's disease and much more commonly in pseudoxanthoma elasticum. Radiologically, both lytic and sclerotic phases are recognized: the lytic phase may be well defined in the calvarium of the skull and is then called osteoporosis circumscripta.

51 B C D

Creutzfeldt-Jakob disease (CJD), Gerstmann-Straussler-Sheinker disease (GSSD), familial fatal insomnia and Kuru are all examples of transmissible spongiform encephalopathies occurring in humans. Bovine spongiform encephalopathy (BSE) occurs in cattle and scrapie in sheep. GSSD is familial, usually of cerebellar onset and tends to have a slower progression than CJD. The spongiform encephalopathies are thought to be due to an

135

abnormal prion protein (PrP) which does not contain nucleic acid but is transmissible. SSPE is produced by a conventional paramyxovirus and PML by a papova virus.

52 A

Precipitating antibodies may give support to the diagnosis but can occur in the absence of disease. Symptoms occur a few hours after exposure and the onset is over weeks or months. Rheumatoid factor is not a feature of extrinsic allergic alveolitis.

53 A B C D

Pancytopenia may be caused by folic acid deficiency as noted in intensive care units and pregnancy. When caused by paroxysmal nocturnal haemoglobinuria it may terminate in aplastic anaemia. In AML both crowding out and inhibition of normal haemopoiesis occur. Haemosiderosis does not produce aplasia except that occurring in terminal sideroblastic anaemia.

54 A B C D E

Other causes of bilateral facial weakness include fascioscapular humeral dystrophy and polymyositis. A unilateral basal pontine lesion may produce an ipsilateral lower motor neurone seventh cranial nerve palsy due to involvement of the upper motor neurone fibres which subsequently cross to the contralateral seventh cranial nerve nucleus. An associated contralateral hemiplegia will usually be evident (Millard-Gubler syndrome). Bilateral lesions above the pons can produce bilateral upper motor neurone facial weakness, pseudobulbar palsy and associated long tract signs.

55 B D E

Pleural effusions are very unusual in PCP. In asbestos related disease, effusions are frequently benign. Blood staining may be due to a PE or malignancy.

56 B C D

Erythropoietin (EPO) is a 30 kD glycoprotein produced in the single isoform by the kidney, and in foetal life, the liver. The liver continues to produce small amounts of endogenous EPO even in anephric adults. Anaemia or hypoxia stimulate EPO production and it acts on the bone marrow to increase red cell production selectively. Recombinant erythropoietin therapy in renal failure can exacerbate hypertension and is associated with increased risk of seizures.

57 C

A is false, r is simply the correlation coefficient. B is false, there is a positive association between the two variables. D is false, a statistically significant correlation does not necessarily imply a causal relationship. E is false, the small value of p implies that the mathematical relationship present has been established as statistically significant, so more than sufficient infants were studied.

58 A C E

It is important to look for treatable causes of dementia. Treatable causes include B12, folic acid or thiamine deficiency, normal pressure hydrocephalus, Wilson's disease, cerebral syphilis and cerebral neoplasms.

59 A D E

The genetic code is carried by nuclear DNA which consists of two complementary strands. Series of three nucleotides (bases: adenosine, cytosine, thymidine and guanine) on one strand code for each amino acid and also provide codes for stopping and starting transcription. In RNA, thymidine is replaced by uracil. Transcription is the process of transferring genetic code from DNA to RNA. DNA consists of exons containing genetic material and introns of apparently functionless nucleotide sequences which are not transcribed into mature messenger RNA. Southern blotting is a semi-quantitative method for measuring DNA in chromatographic gels and Northern blotting is used to measure RNA. Endonucleases are enzymes (mostly derived from micro-organisms) which digest DNA, cutting it at specific nucleotide sequences, allowing detection of small mutations given appropriate complementary DNA probes. DNA polymerase is an enzyme used to replicate significant amounts of DNA from tiny samples for research and diagnosis (forensic DNA fingerprinting, prenatal genetic diagnosis from chorionic villus biopsy etc).

60 E

HIV-positive patients with tuberculosis respond well to standard combination therapy. Although multiple drug resistance (MDR TB) has been a particular problem in this group it is not host dependent and fatal cases of MDR TB have occurred in previously healthy hospital staff. Standard treatment is now 6 months rifampicin and isoniazid with pyrazinamide for the first two months. In spinal disease the initial site of infection is the intervertebral disc.

RECOMMENDED READING AND REFERENCE BOOKS

You will need to have easy access to a comprehensive general medical textbook, which should provide adequate detail for most background reading in the subject areas represented in these practice exams. However, some subjects require more detailed specialist texts and a separate reading list is provided below. The final answer to some questions which may arise in everyday practice may not be found even in the largest general medical textbook. The examples of larger specialist texts and in some cases smaller reference texts are widely available. However, if that particular reference text is not available in your library, there will almost certainly be an adequate substitute. There are also numerous shorter textbooks on individual subjects (e.g. Lecture Notes series) which are invaluable for quick reference when working in a specialist area. However, by the time you have bought a few of these, you may already have spent what it would cost to buy a comprehensive general medical textbook; this may be more valuable to you in the long term.

Be aware that there are differences between textbooks and some subjects go out of date more rapidly than others (e.g. Pharmacology). In particular, American texts express different views when compared with their British counterparts, particularly in the areas of diagnosis, management and therapeutics. American texts may also be confusing because they do not use SI units.

Although it is more relevant to the second part of the MRCP examination, getting into the habit of reading the leading articles, editorials and key papers in the general medical journals is a very useful way of keeping up to date (*BMJ, Lancet, British Journal of Hospital Medicine, New England Journal of Medicine*). In addition, the Medicine International series is a widely used revision aid, as the articles are structured for this purpose. The 'rolling' contents ensures that this series is usually very up to date.

General medical reference texts
Weatherall D J, **Oxford Textbook of Medicine**, 3rd edition, Oxford University Press, 1995.
Harrison T R, **Principles of Internal Medicine**, 13th edition, McGraw Hill, 1994.
Wyngaarden J B & Loeb R F, **Cecil's Textbook of Medicine**, 19th edition, Saunders, 1991.

Shorter general medical texts
Edwards C R W & Bouchier I A D, **Principles and Practice of Medicine,** 4th edition, Blackwell Scientific, 1991.
Kumar P J & Clarke M L, **Clinical Medicine**, 5th edition, Ballière, 1994.
Rubenstein D & Wayne D, **Lecture Notes on Clinical Medicine**, 4th edition, Blackwell Scientific, 1991.

Specialist text books
Basic sciences
Ganong W, **Review of Medical Physiology**, 17th edition, Appleton Lange, 1995.
Williams PL, **Gray's Anatomy**, 38th edition, Churchill Livingstone, 1995.
Easterbrook P, **Basic Sciences for the MRCP Part 1**, Churchill Livingstone, 1994.

Cardiology
Julian DG et al, **Diseases of the Heart**, 2nd edition, Ballière, 1995.

Clinical chemistry
Marshall W, **Clinical Chemistry**, 2nd edition, Gower, 1992.
Williams DL & Marks V, **Principles of Clinical Biochemistry**, 2nd edition, Butterworth Heinemann, 1988.

Dermatology
Rook A & Chapman RH, **Textbook of Dermatology**, 5th edition, Blackwell.
Buxton PK, **ABC of Dermatology**, 2nd edition, BMJ, 1993.

Diabetes
Pickup JC & Williams G, **Diabetes**, Blackwell Scientific, 1991.
Tattersall RB & Gale EAH, **Diabetes: Clinical Management**, Churchill Livingstone, 1990.

Endocrinology
Grossman A, **Clinical Endocrinology**, Blackwell Scientific, 1992.
Besser GM et al, **Fundamentals of Clinical Endocrinology**, 2nd edition, Gower, 1994.

Gastroenterology
Sherlock S & Dooley J, **Diseases of the Liver and Biliary System**, 9th edition, Blackwell, 1992.
Sleisinger MH & Fordtran JS, **Gastrointestinal Disease**, 5th edition, Saunders, 1993.

Genetics
Mueller RF & Young ID, **Elements of Medical Genetics**, 9th edition, Churchill Livingstone, 1995.

Haematology
Hoffbrand AV & Lewis JE, **Postgraduate Haematology**, 3rd edition, Heinemann, 1989.
Hoffbrand AV & Pettitt JE, **Essential Haematology**, 3rd edition, Blackwell Scientific, 1992.

Immunology
Haeney M & Chapel H, **Essentials of Clinical Immunology**, 3rd edition, Blackwell Scientific, 1993.

Recommended Reading and Reference Books

Infectious diseases
Mandel GL et al, **The Principles and Practice of Infectious Diseases**, 4th edition, Churchill Livingstone, 1994.
Adler MW, **ABC of AIDS**, 3rd edition, BMJ, 1993.

Metabolic disorders
Scriver CR, **Metabolic Basis of Inherited Disease**, 7th edition, McGraw Hill, 1994.

Neurology
Walton Sir J, **Brains Diseases of the Nervous System**, 10th edition, Oxford University Press, 1993.
Bannister Sir R, **Brains Clinical Neurology**, 7th edition, Oxford University Press, 1992.

Pharmacology and therapeutics
Laurence DR & Bennet PN, **Clinical Pharmacology**, 7th edition, Churchill Livingstone, 1992.
Goodman L & Gilman A, **Pharmacological Basis of Therapeutics**, 9th edition, McGraw Hill, 1996.
Martindale W & Reynolds JEF, **The Extra Pharmacopeia**, 30th edition, The Pharmacological Press, 1993.

Psychiatry
Gelder MG et al, **Oxford Textbook of Psychiatry**, 2nd edition, Oxford University Press, 1989.

Respiratory disease
Seaton A et al, **Crofton & Douglas Respiratory Diseases**, 4th edition, Blackwell Scientific, 1989.
Brewis RAL et al, **Respiratory Medicine**, 2nd edition, Baillère Tindall, 1995.

Rheumatology
Klippel JH & Dieppe PA, **Rheumatology**, Gower, 1994.
Maddison PJ et al, **The Oxford Textbook of Rheumatology**, Oxford University Press, 1993.

Statistics
Bradford Hill A, **A Short Textbook of Medical Statistics**, revised edition, Edward Arnold, 1991.
Pipkin FB, **Medical Statistics Made Easy**, Churchill Livingstone, 1991.
Gardner MJ & Altman DG, **Statistics with Confidence**, BMJ, 1989.
Swinscow TDV, **Statistics at Square One**, 9th edition, BMA, 1995.

MCQs LISTED BY SUBJECT AREA

For those candidates who like to revise subject by subject using our suggested reading and reference list, the following lists of MCQs classified by subject may be of assistance in covering specific subject areas. (Many MCQs combine two subject areas and are therefore listed under more than one category.) The first number denotes which practice exam is referred to, the following number is the question number.

E.g.   3.43 = Practice Exam 3, question number 43.

Basic sciences
1.01 1.23 1.24 1.37 1.42
2.09 2.11 2.12 2.25 2.27
2.30 2.32 2.46 2.49 3.01
3.02 3.08 3.15 3.20 3.26
3.36 3.40 3.43 3.59 4.12
4.17 4.29 4.30 4.35 4.38
4.57 4.58 5.18 5.19 5.20
5.22 5.32 5.37 5.38 5.39
5.40 5.48 5.56

Cardiology
1.10 1.15 1.18 1.31 1.32
1.34 1.43 1.51 1.55 1.58
2.06 2.22 2.31 2.36 2.37
2.44 2.58 3.12 3.31 3.32
3.56 4.08 4.14 4.18 4.19
4.30 4.44 4.52 5.05 5.13
5.29 5.38 5.47

Clinical Pharmacology
1.19 1.40 1.43 1.44 1.51
1.58 2.07 2.19 2.20 2.28
2.31 2.32 2.37 2.38 2.39
2.41 3.07 3.09 3.10 3.18
3.22 3.29 3.57 4.03 4.14
4.16 4.19 4.26 4.53 5.09
5.14 5.24 5.35 5.36 5.39
5.40 5.44 5.48

Dermatology
1.07 1.57 2.55 3.46 4.41
5.02

Endocrinology
1.12 1.21 1.30 1.42 1.45
2.09 2.18 2.33 2.60 3.08
3.20 3.23 3.40 3.50 3.59
4.04 4.20 4.31 4.35 4.46
4.55 5.07 5.16 5.25 5.41

Gastroenterology
1.11 1.13 1.22 1.32 1.44
1.56 2.01 2.10 2.20 2.28
2.41 3.10 3.17 3.25 3.33
3.51 4.06 4.13 4.31 4.47
4.53 4.54 4.56 5.08 5.17
5.27 5.30 5.35 5.39

Genetics
1.04 1.28 1.59 2.33 2.52
2.59 3.43 3.48 5.04 5.34
5.42 5.59

Haematology
1.14 1.29 1.38 1.41 1.46
1.52 2.02 2.26 2.29 2.34
2.40 3.02 3.16 3.22 3.24
3.30 3.49 3.52 3.57 4.21
4.27 4.48 4.58 5.09 5.15
5.33 5.42 5.53

Infectious Diseases and AIDS
1.05 1.08 1.11 1.20 1.35
1.40 1.47 1.57 2.08 2.23
2.35 2.53 3.03 3.13 3.25
3.37 3.44 3.53 3.58 4.06
4.09 4.21 4.22 4.32 4.39
4.42 4.54 5.15 5.17 5.29
5.30 5.43 5.49 5.60

Immunology
1.23 1.37 2.11 2.46 2.55
3.01 4.41 4.57 5.18 5.37

Metabolism and Diabetes
1.03 1.16 1.19 1.24 1.31
1.38 1.39 1.42 1.48 2.04
2.19 2.27 2.36 3.09 3.17
3.18 3.21 3.26 3.54 4.04
4.05 4.13 4.23 4.49 4.50
5.11 5.26 5.34 5.44 5.50

Nephrology
1.25 1.41 1.59 2.07 2.29
3.03 3.19 3.20 3.26 3.39
3.40 3.49 4.12 4.15 4.45
4.49 4.59 5.20 5.36 5.56

Neurology
1.06 1.09 1.17 1.28 1.33
1.36 1.49 1.53 2.04 2.05
2.13 2.16 2.21 2.22 2.24
2.39 2.43 2.45 2.48 2.54
2.57 3.06 3.07 3.11 3.14
3.27 3.35 3.38 3.44 3.45
3.48 3.55 4.02 4.07 4.10
4.22 4.24 4.28 4.34 4.40
4.43 4.51 5.01 5.04 5.06
5.12 5.23 5.28 5.31 5.46
5.51 5.54 5.58

Ophthalmology
1.33 3.54 3.58 4.55 5.11

Psychiatry
1.03 1.26 2.14 2.17 2.45
2.51 3.04 3.07 3.42 4.03
4.10 4.26 4.37 4.60 5.21
5.24 5.31 5.58

Respiratory Disease
1.08 1.27 1.47 1.50 1.54
1.60 2.15 2.25 2.38 2.42
2.47 2.56 2.59 3.05 3.15
3.28 3.34 3.36 3.37 3.47
4.01 4.11 4.25 4.29 4.33
4.42 4.52 5.03 5.22 5.32
5.45 5.52 5.55

Rheumatology
1.29 1.48 2.03 3.01 3.53
5.10 5.50

Statistics
1.02 2.50 3.41 4.36 5.57

INDEX

Index

Drug interaction 1.43
Drug side effects 4.3
Duchenne muscular dystrophy 2.52, 5.4
Dust diseases 1.54
Dysarthria 5.12
Dysphasia 5.12
Dystrophia myotonica 3.48

E. coli 3.25
E Antigen 1.11
ECG 1.18, 1.55, 3.12, 4.3, 4.14, 4.18, 5.5, 5.29, 5.47
Ectopic ACTH 3.34
EEG 2.45, 3.27, 5.31
EMG 2.16, 5.4
Emphysema 4.25, 5.32
Enalapril 1.51, 5.36
Enalaprilat 5.40
Encephalitis 4.22
Encephalopathy 2.13
Endocarditis 3.2, 5.29, 5.43
Endonucleases 5.19, 5.59
Endothelin-1 3.40
Endothelium derived relaxation factor 4.30
Enterohepatic recirculation 5.39
Enzyme induction 2.32, 3.29
Enzyme inhibitors 5.40
Eosinophilia 1.47, 3.19, 3.28, 5.49
Eosinophils 5.37
Epilepsy 1.34, 2.5, 3.35
Erb's muscular dystrophy 1.4
Erythema nodosum 3.47
Erythroblasts 4.21
Erythromycin stearate 3.10
Erythropoietin 5.56
Ethinyloestradiol 5.39
Exophthalmos 4.55
Extrinsic allergic alveolitis 5.52
Extrinsic alveolar lavage 2.25

Familial polyposis coli 1.4
Farmer's lung 3.28, 4.1
Femoral nerve 4.40
Fenofibrate 2.19
Ferritin 1.38
Fibrin degradation products 2.2
Fibrosing alveolitis 1.37, 3.36, 4.25, 4.33
Finasteride 5.40
First pass metabolism 1.44
Flucytosine 3.44
Folate 3.16
Fungal 3.53

G Proteins 4.35
G6PD deficiency 3.57
GABA 3.7, 4.26
Gait 4.51

Galactorrhoea 2.28
Gallstones 2.10
Gastrin 4.31
Gaucher's disease 3.43
Gene 3.43
Gene therapy 2.59
Genetic 5.59
Gentamicin 1.44, 2.7
Giant cell arteritis 2.3
Giardiasis 4.56
Gilbert's syndrome 2.10
Glaucoma 5.11
Glibenclamide 3.9
Glipizide 1.19
Glomerulonephritis 1.25, 5.29
Glucagon 2.18
Glucogenolysis 2.18
Gluconeogenesis 2.18, 3.9
Glucose 1.16, 1.19
Glucuronide conjugates 4.53
Gluten sensitivity 1.22
Glyceryl trinitrate 1.32, 2.7
Gnathostomiasis 3.58
Gold 1.25
Gonococcal 1.40
Goodpasture 4.45
Gout 3.24
Graves' disease 4.55
Growth factors 4.58
Guillain-Barré syndrome 4.22, 5.54
Gynaecomastia 3.50, 4.19

Haemarthrosis 1.29
Haemoglobin F 5.42
Haemolysis 4.12
Haemolytic anaemia 2.34, 3.57
Haemophilia A 4.48
Haemophilia B 1.29, 2.52
Haemosiderosis 5.53
Haloperidol 2.39
Ham's acid lysis test 3.49
Hantavirus 3.13
HDL 1.24
Headache 4.47
Heart disease, ischaemic 1.24
Heart sound 2.44
Helicobacter pylori 5.17
Helminths 1.47
Hemianopia 5.12
Hemiplegia 1.17, 1.33, 1.49, 2.22, 4.24, 5.46
Heparin 2.2, 5.9
Hepatic cirrhosis 1.44
Hepatic coma 3.22
Hepatic encephalopathy 5.27
Hepatitis B 1.11, 2.1, 4.6
Hepatitis C 4.6, 4.54, 5.30
Hepatitis D 1.11, 4.6

Index

Index